Ten Fat Loss Prescriptions For
Hard Working Achievers
Lose 20-100 Lbs, Gain Energy & Feel Healthy Again!

I0842242

THE
12 HOUR
SHIFT

SLIMDOWN

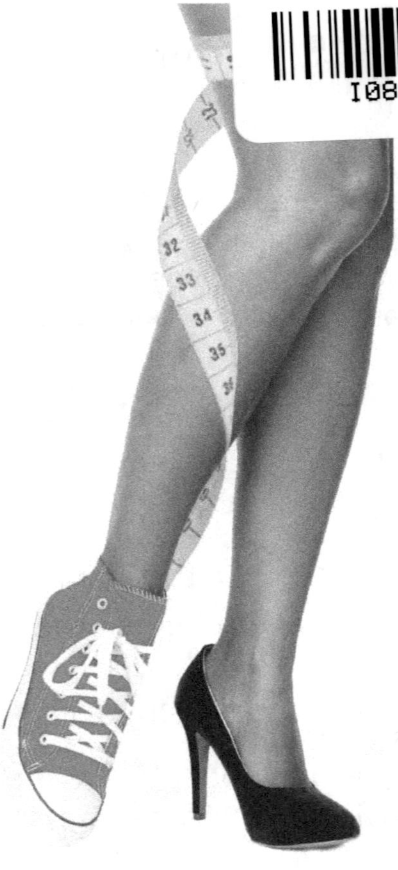

SYLVIA WILLIAMS

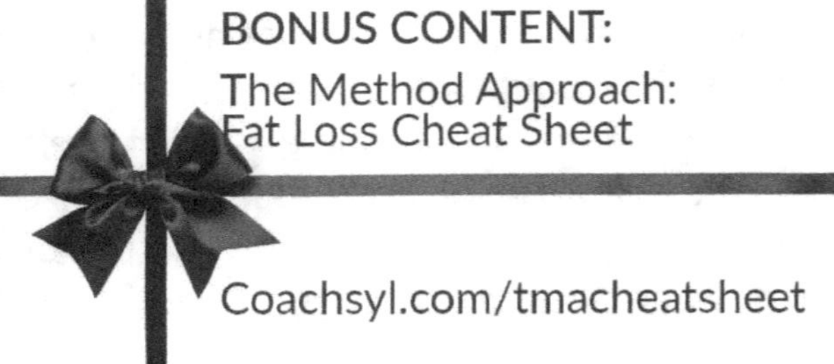
BONUS CONTENT:
The Method Approach:
Fat Loss Cheat Sheet

Coachsyl.com/tmacheatsheet

Cover Design: Hammad Khalif
Page Design: Sarco Press
Chief Editor: Terence O'Connor
Copy Editor: Carol Bettencourt

Disclaimer:

This book is not intended to be a substitute for the medical advice of a licensed physician. The reader should consult with their doctor in any matters relating to his/her health.

The author has made every effort to ensure that accuracy of the information within this book was correct at time of publi-cation. The author does not assume and hereby disclaims any liability to any party for any loss, damage, or disruption caused by errors or omissions, whether such errors or omissions result from accident, negligence, or any other cause.

To a man who is everything God desired me to have. Some call him Ron, but I call him my rock. Thank you for allowing me to do all of the crazy things my heart desires and to fuel my passion for helping and serving women the best way I know how. If people knew you the way that I do they would love you the way that I do, unconditionally.

Forever

Ronlvia

I also dedicate this book to all of my 'Finish Getters'! Your continued commitment to transforming your life through health and fitness has not gone unnoticed.

Finish Getter

[Fin·ish Get·ter]

A person coached by Syl that starts his or her journey with the end in mind to reach his or her desired goal.

ACKNOWLEDGMENTS

My mission is to create an image with words of the people that helped me become the woman that I am: Christian, Wife, Mother, G-Mama, Daughter, Sister, and Sheep.

Lord, you are my strength. Ron, you are my rock. Marcell, Taylor, and Ryan, you are my heart. Aslan, you have my heart. Mama, you are my world. Twyana, Tameisha, and Nicole you are my blood, and it runs thicker than water. Pastor Robb and Mrs. Linda, you are my teachers. I believe this day would have never come without you in my life. I am forever grateful!

To my Daddy, Grandmother, Aunts, Uncles, Daughter-in-law, cousins, sister and brothers-in-law: Just as Noah had help building the Ark, my life was influenced, touched and molded by all of you. Thank you forever!

And to the many people who inspired this book for their honest feedback and wise advice, a huge "Thank you."

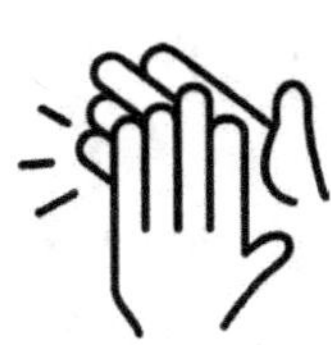

"I have had the pleasure and great opportunity to have received guidance and support from a strong woman who is committed to helping others find their own unique path to health and fitness through mindful eating and exercise, Coach Syl.

This is not an easy task as anyone who is reading this book can appreciate. It is especially difficult when you are struggling with a busy schedule, responsibilities and time constraints. I understand this because I have been a nurse and now nurse practitioner for many years. In my opinion, it is one of the hardest professions to achieve a fair balance between your home life and work responsibilities.

Likely the biggest reason for this is that we (nurses) seem to automatically put everyone and everything else before ourselves. It is very easy to talk yourself out of going to the gym when you are exhausted. It is also very hard to find time to sit down to have a healthy lunch and sometimes even a bathroom break for crying out loud when you still have patient care documentation to complete.

Making a commitment to finding the time is one key. Most nurses are masters at prioritizing and multitasking when it comes to taking care of everyone else, but weight loss and overall well-being comes when there is time set aside to take care of ourselves."

Therese Roche, APRN-BC

"Being a nurse, I am responsible for teaching people about their "health" on a daily basis. But sometimes you can lose sight of how to do that for yourself! You find yourself needing a catalyst. Coach Syl is THAT person. She is dedicated, driven and genuinely cares about the health of her clients. She is a living testament to strategies that work. This book is a must-read if you want to "find your way." Enjoy! And Congratulations Sylvia! You continue to amaze and inspire me!"

Kristine J. Bobbitt, RN, BSN

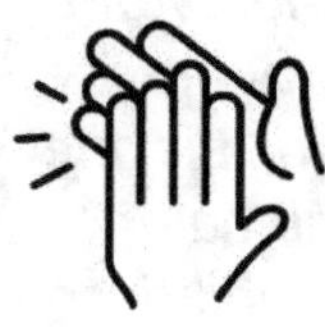

"Coach Syl is the most influential, innovative black woman I've come to know. She's encouraging, informative and non- judgmental making every effort possible to make you feel warm, welcomed and accepted.

My most touching experience was when she reached out to me over the phone out of thousands I'm sure to have a 1:1 conversation about my goals. As an RN with 26 yrs. of experience this is the first weight loss coach that ever empathizes with me and truly understands the plight of the nurse; eating habits and weight loss."

Ms. Lenell Davis-Johnson RN BSN

"Finally a guidebook that affirms it's not all about counting calories and spending hours in the gym. Who has time for that? I agree with Coach Syl that every nurse, or in my case Dental Hygienist needs these Prescriptions—and strategies. The ideas expressed in this book are long overdue. The Golden book for the scrub wearing woman. Thank you, Coach Syl."

Karen Gwartzman, RDH and Bestselling Author

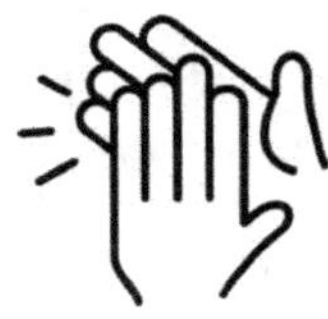

",, I was coached by Sylvia, and within the first seven days, I had improvements in my health and weight. Her program is the real deal, and after reading the 12 Hour Shift, you will have a proven system that will get you the health results you have been trying to achieve. In the words of Coach Syl, "Just Trust The Process!"

Rakisha Sloane, Ed. D.

"Coach Syl has practical experience to share to motivate and direct you straight to seeing results. If you follow her tried and true system you will feel better, be healthier, and start to shed those pounds. You will also want to stick with it because the steps are simple. She encourages accountability and setting goals. I found myself responding to the expectation that my dreams could be reached!"

Jane Jarosz M.S., OTR/L, LMT

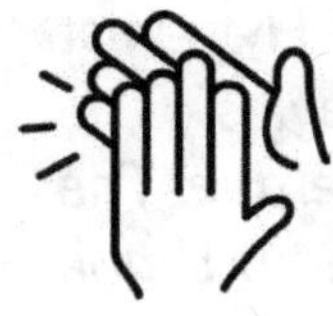

"Because there is so much trendy hype about weight loss, it is essential that the real value of these recommendations be spoken loudly as Coach Syl has done in this book. As a nurse who once endured the treacherous 12 - 16-hour shifts, I can say a road map such as this would have saved significant pain in my life. Treat yourself to this bold yet friendly guide, with easy and practical steps to improve your health, and nourish all of who you are and will be."

Dr. Debbie Karas, APN-BC, RN

CONTENTS

INTRODUCTION

Hey! I'm back!

Even though it hasn't been that long since I first wrote this book, it's time for a brand new version. The need to get this message into more hands came sooner, rather than later. As usual, when I get really excited about something, I just couldn't help myself! Over and over again, with client after client, I find that the ideas in this book really do work. I want to share them with as many people as possible, because I know what a tremendous difference the right approach to weight loss can make. This isn't about just a physical transformation. It's about a life transformation.

Originally, I wrote this book especially for nurses. Over the years, I have had a high percentage of nurses in my program, and I've always had a special place in my heart for them. They obviously know health, but long hours and junk food on the run between patient checks is not a great prescription for maintaining a healthy weight.

However, I discovered that nurses are not the only ones working long shifts and facing weight loss challenges. All kinds of people work shifts that are well beyond an eight-hour work day. Whether you are a beautician, an entrepreneur, a factory worker, hospitality worker or even a truck driver, you may find yourself facing long shifts. Whether you are on your feet, at a computer or behind the wheel, you may be at work for way too long!

How are those fourteen-hour days working for you? How many of your meals are grab-it-and-go junk food? Is sleep deprivation your major form of exercise? Do you ache, and not in a good way, from standing too long or sitting too long, or just working too long, period?

With this revised version of my book, I wanted to extend my message to all dedicated, hard-working, high-achievers. You may have a busy career, a busy home life, or both. By every measure, you do very well in life, but fitness is a real challenge. You're willing to take on those long shifts or extra hours to provide for your family, but what about you?

Sometimes, the problem is that after taking care of others – whether patients, clients, customers or co-workers, not to mention family – we often leave little room for taking care of ourselves. And, even when we do carve out the time and energy for ourselves, weight loss is a challenge.

Solid evidence points to just how prevalent the problem is. According to an article in healthline.com, truckers are the most overweight group by profession, with others who work long shifts, including police, firefighters, nurses and orderlies not far behind. In fact, according to the Center for Disease Control, 36.5% of adults in the United States are obese. Obesity is defined as a Body Mass Index of 30 or higher, which is around 180 lbs. for someone who is 5'5". Even if you are not obese, if you are overweight, you could be headed in that direction.

Let's examine exactly what these statistics mean. At first glance, they seem to mean that there are a whole lot of people who need extra-large clothes and who just don't look as fit and stylish as they might if they dropped twenty, fifty or even a hundred pounds. Maybe you are too busy working to really be concerned about style or fitness.

But, the problem is much more serious than that. The CDC states that obesity is related to some of the leading causes of preventable death, including heart disease, Type 2 Diabetes, stroke and certain types of cancer. Doctors concur, and the American Medical Association has classified obesity as a disease, with numerous health repercussions. There are serious economic repercussions as well. The National League of Cities reports that on average, obesity results in direct costs of $50 million per every 100,000 people in cities with the highest obesity rates. As the statistics show, weight problems affect many of us, especially those of us with work shifts that extend well beyond a typical eight-hour day. This is especially troubling to me, because I know that as you put in that extra time, you have your heart set on doing good things, not on creating life threatening health issues or economic burdens. Even in the health care professions, where practitioners should, and do, "know better," there are problems with weight and fitness.

Enter me. I have walked in those same shoes. I am a hard-working, high achieving woman. I was advising my clients about the dangers of obesity when I was 50 lbs. overweight! Emphasis on WAS.

Finally, I said, "enough." Since then, my journey has been amazing, though not always smooth. But I have done it, and I can offer legitimate, workable advice to help you do it too.

This book is not full of the typical hype, such as "7 Ways to Lose 10 Pounds in one Day!" You might not think that's such a bad idea, but I happen to know that it just won't work. Sorry, folks, that's the way it is. Most of the advice on the internet about weight loss is just fluff, designed to rank high in searches, but not carefully researched to be of any real help.

This book offers a direct approach to a serious topic, based on experience and feedback. If you are willing to tackle the goal of weight loss just as seriously as you have taken on your other life goals, then you deserve resources that can really help you.

Here, based on my own personal experience and the experiences of my clients, are my ten prescriptions every hard working woman - and man - needs to get back into those favorite clothes. No more "fat pants." It is time for your "boss pants!" Instead of theory, mantras or navel contemplation, I provide you with real-life tips, tricks, and tools that work.

Are you ready?

Let's do it!

CHAPTER
1

DISCOVER YOUR
WHY PRESCRIPTION

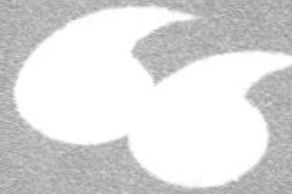

"What you get by achieving your goals is not as important as what you become by achieving your goals."

Zig Ziglar

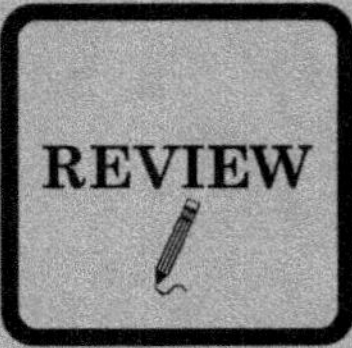

"Last year, I finally had enough of being unhappy about my weight. I was either going to lose it or start seeing a therapist to learn to accept my body as it was. Coach Syl's challenge was my last chance and became my best decision.

I would joke that working out was going to give me a heart attack, but at least someone would call 911. Frankly, that was a better option than the possibility of having a heart attack while sitting at home on the couch, which was a real possibility, given my sedentary lifestyle and poor nutrition.

But it didn't kill me, it made me stronger. And in time my breathless panting "I can't" became purposeful, relaxed, deep-breathing into "Yes, I can."

Success during the challenge lead me to more weight loss success through the holidays, and on and on. Since joining, I've lost more than 50 pounds and found happiness and contentedness with my body and a feeling of confidence I've never known."

—Client

Your *Why* can help you lose weight!

Signing up for the latest fitness craze or the newest weight loss program is usually very exciting. Just the thought of being able to get back into those smaller clothes buried in the back of your drawer would be a dream come true! Have you ever tried to do that?

I remember attempting to squeeze into an old pair of "too small" jeans before the start of a new program to get inspired. I thought it would be a great way to get a reading on how far I had to go. I wiggled. I squeezed. I jumped. And, I sighed. There was no way those jeans were going on my body, or even mostly over my legs, without busting a vein!

Isn't this the type of foolish thing we do when we're starting at a new gym or working out with a new trainer? Our head really gets in the game. We pump ourselves up and start to truly believe anything is possible, even losing that stubborn fat that sits comfortably just below the bra strap. You know what I'm talking about. We call it "bra fat."

Now be honest, all my ladies reading this book, isn't that one of the first places you look to see if that crazy diet plan is working. Heck, if you can get rid of bra fat surely you can burn the rest of it.

As we start to get our game on, we do – and buy - all the right things. The weekend before, you may begin to prep and portion your food or buy that new fancy water bottle. You may set up an account on MyFitnessPal, and just to show the world how serious you are about this new quest, a shiny, new purple Fitbit makes a home on your wrist.

It seems like you are invincible, but then, faster than you could say "Biggest Loser," you've already fallen off the wagon. Has this ever happened to you?

It happens to a lot of people. I call it the battle of the "3's". Most people fall off the wagon by the third day, third week or third month. I believe that happens when we start the journey with unrealistic expectations and a false sense of hope.

False Sense of Hope

Let me explain. You may put your hope and trust in a program, counting on the advertised results, only to be disappointed. The disappointment has nothing to do with the quality of the program or its record of success. It has nothing to do with the trainer. The problem comes from where you put your hope. What exactly are you hoping to accomplish by losing weight? What even makes it worth trying to do?

Think about it, when a person tells friends and family that they are getting married, one of the first questions is, "Why do you want to marry this person?" No one starts by asking, "Do you think it's going to last?" At least I hope that's not the first question. If it is, I would call that a RED FLAG! ;) Of course, you think it will last, because you have a deep, personal connection to the person you are marrying and explaining that connection explains your why.

The "Why" Concept

For lots of people, "why" is a hard concept. It isn't as tangible as the new water bottle or hard numbers like your weight or dress size. So, what exactly is it?

Let's break down the mechanics of discovering your Why. Start by asking yourself a series of questions that will cause you to look deep into your soul. At first glance, these questions will seem predictable and common. And, as you answer them, you may need to dig a few layers deeper with each one. Trust me though, once you dig deep enough, you will know that you have found your why. Reaching those deep level answers ultimately determines your victory.

These answers compel you to make a real effort of time and energy. They help you make the changes needed to see real results. Despite what some people may think, the answers to these questions aren't complicated. In fact, you may find that they are powerfully simple.

Ask yourself:

- *Why do you care what people think about your extra weight?*

- *Why do you want to live a better, healthier, longer life?*

- *Why does it matter what your body looks like?*

Remember to dig deep. If the answer to "Why do you want to lose weight?" is "I want to fit in smaller jeans," ask yourself why that is important. If the answer is "I want a healthier, longer life," again, ask yourself why that is important. Go deep to get to the true why.

The answers to these critical questions form the basis of your weight loss journey. They give you valuable and true insight into your deepest desires – who are you, who do you want to be, and what matters to you. What do you love? What brings you happiness, contentment and security?

Incidentally, the answers to these questions are evolutionary. They will alter, adjust, and evolve as time goes by. Depending on where you are and what you're doing in life, these answers WILL change. As your health journey – and your life journey – bring you closer to the person you are meant to be, you may get even more in touch with your true why. And as circumstances change, your needs and your why may change.

So discovering your why is your most important weight loss tool, but it also gives you valuable insight into what your soul wants and clarity about your life goals. Furthermore, the ultimate answer to your Why, when tied in with your weight loss journey, gives you a clearer, more focused goal to work towards – ultimately yielding better, more definitive results.

As you can see, the process of discovering your Why is actually quite simple if you truly consider it. When you strip away the outside influences, the worries, the judgments, and "good" intentions of the people that surround you, you can easily and readily uncover the answer you're searching for.

Maybe, as you read this, you are beginning to think about your why. Maybe you have even already managed to answer some of the "why" questions and have an idea of your why. If it still isn't clear, don't worry. Often people need to think about this, or even meditate or pray. Some of us are so in tune with the needs of others, or with what the world thinks we should be about, that it takes some real soul searching to find ourselves. Don't give up though. You need an emotional connection to your Why; a clear understanding of why this weight loss journey is important to you at a core level.

Discovering Your "Why"

There are ways to discover your why that go deeper than external circumstances. Here's a powerful tip: Identify all of the times you've attempted to lose weight or get healthy before. Can you remember? Once? Several times? Great, you just identified that each of those times, motivation was not in sync with your Why. If you had an emotional connection to the motivation, or had unearthed the real reason for

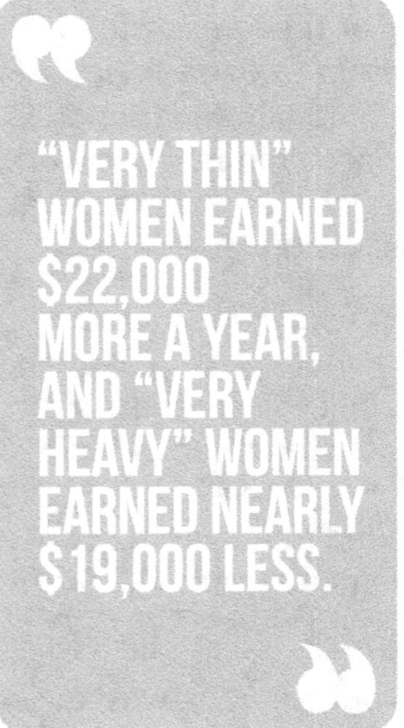

why you wanted to lose the weight or get healthy again you wouldn't be reading this book today.

For example, if you really wanted to lose weight to fit back into your old clothes, attract a mate, or apply for that new job; your Why would be deeper than that. Perhaps, you feel you need approval, acceptance or ...love. But, go a step further.

There's another way to look at your Why. It's by asking yourself, "What would happen if...?" What would happen if your health didn't change? What would happen if you didn't transform your body, lose the weight or get off the medications? There must some reason why you have not asked yourself these questions, or you would have changed a long time ago. However, to truly be satisfied with yourself, you must be honest with yourself.

Often, when a person has a behavior that they should change, but can't, we call that "a monkey on their back." Imagine if you had a monkey on your back and the monkey represented all of the stress and pain you've experienced walking around with the extra weight. For some, that monkey is lost time with family and friends. Others may say the monkey is missed opportunities in the workplace. Whether it is fair or not, how we look and whether we appear fit influences opinions about us and our abilities.

For example, a study published in the Journal of Applied Psychology in 2010 analyzed pay discrepancies between people of different sizes. Dramatic differences were found. The study separated women's body sizes into categories of "very thin," "thin," "average," "heavy," and "very heavy." It found that compared to women of average weight, "very thin" women earned $22,000 more a year, and "very heavy" women earned nearly $19,000 less.

Whether your why includes professional goals or personal goals, the point is that many of us who have struggled with our weight are walking around with these huge monkeys on our backs. The only thing that can get the monkey off your back is coming face to face with your Why. It's like having a come to Jesus moment where you can finally voice what you really want out of life or express how you truly feel about a situation.

You will know exactly when you've discovered your Why because the monkey will vanish and all that will be left is you standing with your shoulders back, and your head held high. It's like when you say, "I just know that I know!" You will know that you've discovered it.

The Power of "Why"

I love it when my clients experience this moment. At the moment, I am thinking of one in particular. She had just completed one of our weight loss challenges, and she met with me to discuss continuing with one of our longer programs. Every time I meet with someone about signing up for the program, I ask this question, "What is your Why?"

She looked at me with a calm face and a slight grin and said, "I don't know." She explained that she had been trying to figure it out because she knew that I would ask her, but for some reason, she was coming up blank. I looked at her with a certain amount of intensity, and I said, "Then this is not the time to sign up for the program." I know many trainers would probably just fall out of their chair over turning a possible paying client away, but I had a different thought about it.

My thought was if she did not know her Why, she would never realize true, lasting transformation. Thankfully a few days later she called me and let me know she had discovered her Why.

I remember getting goosebumps when I heard the conviction in her voice. She went on to lose more than 60 pounds with our program and referred nearly half of her family, who each lost between 30 to 60 pounds themselves.

The moral of that story is you can either start a weight loss journey, or you can start a weight loss journey the right way. My client started right, and that's why she realized a lasting transformation.

The thing about your Why is that it's personal, individual and it's honest; sometimes brutally so.

Often, the main barrier or hindrance that separates us from discovering what it is that we truly desire is our own insecurity.

Most of us are so influenced and impacted by the societal ideal of who we're supposed to be, that we tend to lose sight of who we actually are. If we were to strip away all the expectations, wants, beliefs and opinions, which are bombarded at us and focus on our own beings – individually- then we can easily differentiate what it is that society wants us to achieve and what it is that we want for ourselves.

And that want – that desire that stems from your very core is the answer to your Why.

I want you to shed those preconceived notions of how you should look and behave. Leave them behind and just take stock of who you are and how you appear to be when you envision yourself at your healthiest.

Take note that I didn't mention the word 'fittest' here. That's because I realize that fitness is directly associated with societal standards of beauty which weigh you down and cloud your thoughts. However, health and being healthy is all about your personal, individual well-being which encompasses your mental, social and physical well-being.

So essentially when I ask you to envision and imagine for yourself your own person at your healthiest, I do mean that you include within that picture, your happiness and mental relaxation and stability as well.

Take a moment, close your eyes and create an image in your mind – find one that represents what makes you content, everything that's in control and stable in your life.

Picture the person that you deep down on the inside wish to be – that is the answer to your Why. That person you pictured represents who you truly are and Why you must make this change, start your journey and most importantly FINISH your journey.

Use that, hold on to that- write it out if you feel like it; but whatever you do, don't let go of that image once you've found it. Because not only will that image become the mascot for your health and weight loss journey, it'll be that one saving grace which will always bring you back from the brink – from any deviation, back straight on the right path.

I mention deviation from your journey because we're human. Our entire being can sometimes be controlled by our emotions. Emotion can make things happen that we don't want to happen.

Discovering your Why is hands down the most powerful weight loss tool known to man. Without it, you're simply using willpower, and that just won't cut it. How do I know willpower doesn't work? Well, I've tried it at least two dozen times. Don't get me wrong. Yes, people successfully lose weight without going through the process described in this chapter. But, I almost guarantee that their process was a painful one.

Hold on to the "Why"

When we're on a lifestyle change for better health, the process is not easy because there are so many things along the way, which knock us off our path. However, when we have an image – a wholesome goal to anticipate and work towards, we're better able to control our journey. We can successfully navigate the twists and turns and stay on course.

I know that some of what I have covered might seem a little fuzzy. That's why I've prepared a prescription filled with tips and tricks that you can use as a compass.

Not sure where to start? Let's make a plan together!
You can scan the QR Code for quick access to our website.

COACH SYL'S ℞

THINK OF THE FUTURE

All of us are so occupied with our present, everyday lives, we forget to think about what we're setting ourselves up for in the coming years.

The way you live sets the stage for your future. What better way is there to be your better self, than by picturing a better self in the years to come?

However, by being specific when envisioning one's healthiest self in a future setting, we're making our goal a little more tangible. By adding details and tiny specifications, we're making it more real in our minds – and eventually, more

However, by being specific when envisioning one's healthiest self in a future setting, we're making our goal a little more tangible. By adding details and tiny specifications, we're making it more real in our minds – and eventually, more attainable. So think about the future – fill in those blanks with as many details and as much color as you want.

It will only help solidify your drive to work towards it.

PRIORITIZE

When we lose focus in our lives, we tend to flounder and not accomplish many things we should. As I mentioned earlier, we tend to get so lost in our everyday lives, that we lose sight of the future. At the same time, we lose sight of our individuality and ourselves in the present as well.

To figure out what it is that you wish to accomplish in life regarding weight loss and why you want to achieve your goal, you have to put yourself over everything else.

We tend to brush off self-love and self-importance as inconsequential – especially those of us who have empathic senses that rule our lives. For empaths, their main focus almost always remains on others; what they want, feel and desire all take a back seat.

To find any sort of success in your weight loss journey, you have to put yourself first along with others. You'll also need to tune out the opinions of others and stop thinking and worrying about what it is that they want or need all of the time.

Of course, at times that's easier said than done. I discovered that it is effective to routinely ask, "What do I want?" "What makes me happy?" "What is important and essential in my life? When you have the answers to these questions, then you will know what you need to do.

Compartmentalize

The best way to bring back some clarity to your life is to compartmentalize priorities. You can do that mentally, but I prefer entering a list in a journal. Choose the way that makes you comfortable. Note: Be clear in the divisions and compartments you create.

This separation will help you realize the areas of your life which you're satisfied with, and the ones that you plan on changing. Because we're talking about shifting the focus onto our own person, especially regarding weight loss, these compartments can help you decide why you want to lose weight, and also how you would prefer to lose weight.

For example, when you shift the focus onto yourself and take stock of your own health at the moment, you'll realize that you need to lose weight either because you have a physical goal to attain, or a health concern looming over your head. Once you compartmentalize why you want to lose weight, you can also figure out how you want to go about it.

Be Decisive

Indecisiveness is perhaps one of the biggest pitfalls for people struggling on their weight loss journey.

There are things in life that are important and require your attention, things that force you to shift your focus from yourself to others, and their wants and needs.

However, for an effective, healthy, and long-lasting weight loss journey, it's absolutely mandatory that you instill within yourself some decisiveness.

Some people may be tempted to argue that what I'm talking about here is selfishness instead of decisiveness. I disagree.

It's decisiveness to prioritize one's self. When you decide that you are going to do something for the sake of your own betterment, improvement, and longevity, then it's crucial that you do not, under any circumstances allow anything to change your mind, or divert you from your goals, or distract you from your path.

Once you've made a decision – make sure that you give it your all to stick to it.

Plan

Ah! Planning; My favorite activity when on a weight loss journey.

When you want to lose weight, get toned, shed those pounds and become the healthiest version of yourself, you really cannot possibly think that just walking into the gym with no direction no plan whatsoever, just hoping for the best will accomplish anything.

I'll tell you right here, it really will not accomplish anything at all.

When you are on a weight-loss journey, there's exercise, diet, nutrition, journaling, relaxation, and sleep that you have to take care of. How can you possibly ensure that you're focusing on every element and getting it all done if you have no guidance to follow?

Find yourself a mentor, a counselor, a coach, and take their help to devise a plan for your self – one that is realistic, all-encompassing, and thorough.

Having a clear plan will help you map out a trajectory to follow, and also help you stay on track.

And there you have my prescription of tips that will bring the focus back to your life. In confidence, you will certainly find the answer to that all-important Why. That answer is an honest reflection of yourself, and will help you achieve a state of mental and physical well-being.

PROGRESS NOTES

You need to have and emotional connection to really succeed at weight loss. This is your Why.

Your Why lives with you already.

Assignment: Answer these questions:

- What might happen if I don't lose this weight?.

- What do I see when I envision my life as I want it to be?

- Why is weight loss important for achieving that vision? Be honest! It is the only way.

- Picture the person that you deeply want to be. That will lead you to your *Why*.

Sylvia Williams

CHAPTER 2

GO ROGUE PRESCRIPTION

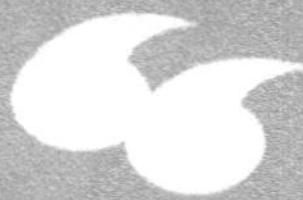

"The only way to keep your health is to eat what you don't want, drink what you don't like, and do what you'd rather not."

Mark Twain

Sylvia Williams

"Last year I started a new role that required me to travel and eat on the road a lot. While I thought I was active because of the constant traveling, I realized the activity did not translate to calorie burning. My eating habits worsened, and I was sitting way too much. I felt...bigger.

Then I weighed myself. Yikes!

I thought, "This scale must be broken." There were 20 more pounds of me. I'm short, and that wasn't good.

I started working out, but I didn't change my eating, and I wasn't eating enough. I took a challenge that literally changed my mindset about weight and diet. Since being part of Coach Syl's program, I have begun shedding those pounds. What I love about her program is the accountability; without it, I would not have been able to keep at it. Huge Thank You, Coach Syl!"

—Client

IT'S TIME TO GO ROGUE!

"Going rogue" has become a popular term for actions that are a bit out of control or off-script. Usually, the person who is going rogue is so compelled to accomplish something that they toss out the normal expected routine. Regardless of their goal, their determination is admirable.

So why in the world would I want you to "go rogue?" The answer is simple.

Your normal routine is not working for you, at least not when it comes to your food habits. It's awfully hard to have even a modest amount of will power when there are yummy temptations everywhere around you. You have enough to do already to reach your goals, so let's not make it even harder by setting up little "food booby-traps" everywhere.

First, you need to clean out your munchy hideouts: cabinets, drawers or closets with hidden stashes of chips, cookies, even leftover Halloween candy. This means everywhere: your kitchen, your bedroom, your desk or workspace, even your car and the bag you take to work.

From a nutritional standpoint, most of us know what is right and what is wrong. So, in this case, "going rogue" means getting rid of all the wrong things. Purge them from your world. If you are not going to eat them, then why would you have them? And if you are going to eat them, well, then you can put this book down right now, since you aren't serious about your weight loss!

Do you feel bad about wasting all that food? Really? You want to save $29.43 worth of junk, but you're willing to risk having to replace your entire wardrobe, run up doctor bills and miss out on life opportunities? I suggest going rogue now!

You think you have enough will power that you can skip this

prescription? Maybe. But how will you feel if you do lose five pounds and then eat the cherry pie? Those five pounds will be right back where they started, on your thighs. I suggest going rogue now!

Speaking from a personal kitchen overhaul experience, it is an amazing feeling to know that there is nothing in your kitchen that can cause you to QUIT your new healthy eating plan. In fact, I don't think I would have written this book had I not gone rogue in my own kitchen.

Take a moment and imagine how you will feel when your cupboards and fridge are full of only good food that can help you. Wouldn't that be better than the roadblocks to your success that you yourself have placed all over your home?

You are about to embark on what could be a fierce struggle between the conniving dirty devil on one shoulder and the supporting angel on the other. The victory takes more than willpower. You must employ tips, tricks, and tools. Make a decision to act, never give up and use every resource at your disposal, including this book.

When it comes to losing weight, you know the drill: Eat less, eat better, move more, rinse and repeat.

Most dieters try using willpower to lose fat. They try to resist the many temptations. I talk more about willpower later on in the book, but the problem of becoming slim by willpower is, it's a 24/7 job, it's never-ending.

Dieting is a pretty miserable experience for most people, butwe're talking about shedding pounds by making changes at home and in the workplace. Most dieters try using will-power to lose fat. They try to resist the many temptations. I talk more about willpower later on in the book, but the problem of becoming slim by willpower is, it's a 24/7 job, it's never-ending.

Dieting is a pretty miserable experience for most people, but we're talking about shedding pounds by making changes at home and workplace.

> WHEN PEOPLE ARE ASKED HOW MANY TIMES A DAY THEY MAKE FOOD DECISIONS, THE AVERAGE GUESS IS 30. THE REAL NUMBER IS CLOSER TO 200.

Simply changing your environment can bring a halt to most mindless eating. I am speaking of eating because you feel like it, rather than because of a conscious decision. When people are asked how many times a day they make food decisions, the average guess is 30. The real number is closer to 200.

Because people are unaware of most of their decisions, they are easily influenced by things around them. Example? The distance of food from their hands or the size of a bowl.

Here are my prescriptions for making kitchen changes that can lead you to eat less. I believe making just one of these changes and sticking with it for at least 21 days will trump any previous results.

Not sure where your extra weight is coming from? Get in touch with Coach Syl at www.coachsyl.com and start accounting for each pound you lose.

COACH SYL'S 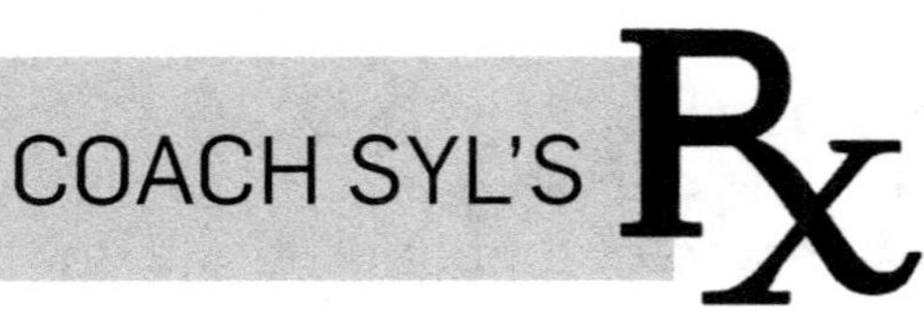

1. De-clutter your kitchen

When participants in one study saw snack foods sitting on the counters of a cluttered and disorganized kitchen, they ate about 44 percent more than people who saw the same snacks in a very neat kitchen.

2. Avoid leaving food out

People who left chips or cookies visible on their kitchen counter weighed about 10 pounds more than people with bare counters, according to one study.

Those who openly displayed breakfast cereal weighed about 21 pounds more, and those who had soft drinks — including diet sodas — on the counter weighed 25 pounds more.

Simply the presence of food is a powerful cue. Every time you pass by a can of soda or a cookie jar you have to ask yourself: Do I want one? After "no," perhaps a "maybe" creeps in. Then "just one" finds its way into the mind game and you lose.

3. Make the kitchen a less appealing hangout

The more time a person spends in their kitchen, the more they tend to eat. So you need to make the kitchen un-inviting, less comfortable. Do you have a little TV on your kitchen counter? If so, get rid of it. Ditto for those comfortable bar stools. Do what you have to do.

4. Put out a fruit bowl

Behold the power of fruit: The person who has a fruit bowl in their house weighs an average of 8 pounds less than their fruitless neighbor.

Out of sight, out of mind is a truism. So is, in sight, in mind. So fill a big bowl with your favorite fruits and put it in a spot people walk by a lot.

5. Foil wrap tempting leftovers in the fridge

People are unlikely to unwrap something in the fridge that is wrapped in aluminum foil. Therefore, you know what kinds of foods to wrap in foil. Conversely, wrap healthy food products in see-through bowls or plastic.

6. Downsize your plates, glasses and utensils

Don't trust yourself to take the right amount of food. If you have 9-inch plates, four ounces of shrimp looks like a lot. The same amount, however, on a 12-inch plate looks like an appetizer and you are tempted to add more.

Downsizing your bowls and plates can make a big difference in the amount of food you eat. Use a 10-inch plate instead of a 12-inch, and you'll likely serve yourself 22 percent less food. Use a tablespoon instead of a big serving spoon; you'll serve about 14 percent less.

7. Hide junk food & other tempting snacks

Stash high-calorie snacks in an inconveniently-placed cupboard — one that's way down low or way up high. So instead of the snacks being spread throughout the kitchen at home, or in the desk drawer right beside you at work, put them all in one off-limits location.

8. SERVE DINNER OFF THE STOVE OR COUNTER

This tip is directed mostly at fast eaters. They often finish first and see the rest of the family still eating, so they have seconds just to keep company with family.

People eat less if serving plates of food are not on the dinner table in front of those eating. Put them on a counter some distance from the dinner table. The diners can still have additional servings, but the inconvenience of going back and forth to the counter tends to result in less food consumption.

PROGRESS NOTES

You can't take a passive approach to dieting and expect any success. Going Rogue is necessary to defend healthy habits. Follow this checklist to make sure you have set the stage for success:

- Remove secret stashes from your house (snack food in your bedside table, Halloween candy in the closet)

- Remove junk food from your desk or work area; avoid areas at work with snacks

- Changing the environment will stop mindless eating

- Declutter the kitchen

- Avoid leaving food out

- Make kitchen a less appealing hang out

- Put out a fruit bowl

- Foil wrap tempting leftovers

- Downsize plates, glasses, and utensils

- Rid your kitchen of secret hideouts of junk food stashes

- Serve dinner off the stove or counter

CHAPTER
3

THE DETOX PRESCRIPTION

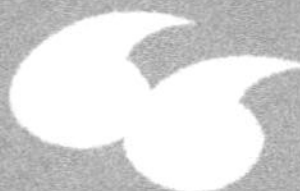

"Start by doing what's necessary; then do what's possible, and suddenly you are doing the impossible."

Francis of Assisi

Sylvia Williams

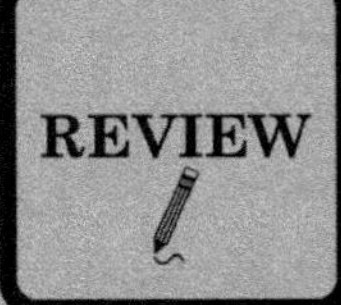

"Before starting my journey, I was hoping and wishing I could lose weight and feel better. I was working too many hours and not taking time for myself. Eating on the run and making bad choices for my health had to stop. I was extremely tired, winded, and could not walk up a flight of stairs without needing to rest afterward. I was on high cholesterol medication, and my blood pressure was creeping higher and higher each year. My health was going in the wrong direction.

I've since reinstated the "Don't give up attitude," which has always been my saving grace. Not only did I do it for my physical health but also for my mental and spiritual health.

Life is short, and I felt a now-or-never urgency! I'm excited to announce that I

- *No longer take cholesterol meds*

- *Can run up a flight of stairs with little effort*

- *Am stronger, feel great and have more energy*

- *Know how to eat, shop for food, prep and PLAN my meals*

- *Dropped 50 pounds! "*

—Client

Keep Them Clean With a Detox!

The word "Them" refers to your liver, kidney, colon, and skin. For example, the liver has its own built-in detox system; it secretes bile and makes protein. That's a pretty big job, and from time-to-time, it needs to get cleaned up and maintained. Detox is the way.

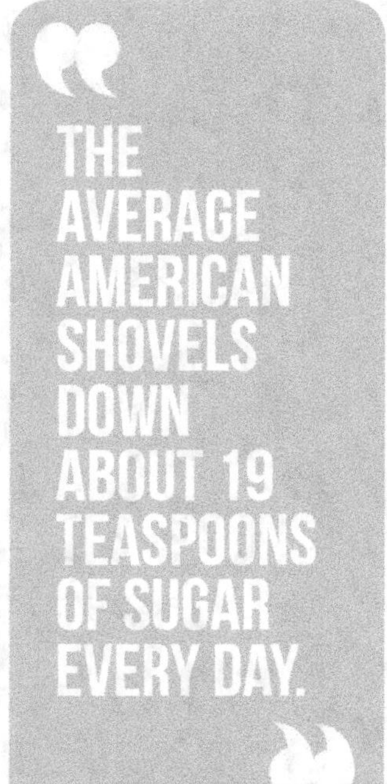

Detox nurses can relate to this Prescription. Detoxing serves many purposes. Many people think a detox facility is only for drug and alcohol addicts. News flash: Sugar addiction leads the pack.

Cocaine is the second-most commonly trafficked drug in the U.S. and kills between 5,000 and 6,000 people. Number one is heroin with just under 12,000 deaths. The two illegal drugs together take about 18,000 lives.

That's a lot. However, there is a single, legal, food product that is responsible for over 25,000 deaths.

The product? Soft drinks. Note: The researchers didn't even look at junk foods that contain processed sugar.

Those findings come from only one of *many* studies that have highlighted the dangers of sugar consumption. It causes plaque that produces cavities. It causes cancer. Sugar is largely to blame for the U.S. obesity epidemic. And yet, the average American shovels down about 19 teaspoons of sugar every day.

HOW TO KICK SUGAR ADDICTION? DETOX.

Detox is often associated with deprivation, hunger, weird foods, juice only diets and colonics. We tend to balance if the "perceived" pain and suffering of detox are worse than the "maybe" dangers of sugar overconsumption.

That argument is bogus. It assumes what is not true. There's a form of detox that's all about fabulous, delicious food. This detox jumpstarts your health and reboots your metabolism. It's enjoyable, easy to do and a direct route to feeling fabulous.

It's what I have my clients do, and you can do it too, in just 14 days.

Over the last several years, I've helped hundreds of clients who suffered from the harmful effects of the wrong foods. In addition to chemical additives, they were ingesting boatloads of sugar and wheat flour; more than 80 pounds of sugar and over 130 pounds of flour per person per year, according to the U.S. Department of Agriculture! This dietary apocalypse not only fostered obesity, it completely derailed their health systems. Moreover, these victims blame themselves for being unable to succeed at controlling their eating habits or cravings.

Millions of us, in fact, over half the population, suffer from what I call FLF Disorder. That's when you Feel Like Fluff, or you have that fluffy feeling. Sometimes it's annoying symptoms such as achy joints or muscles, brain fog, fatigue, headaches, allergies or a bloated stomach, or more serious problems such as autoimmune diseases, migraines, asthma, acne, irritable bowel, reflux, arthritis or worse.

By "detox," I mean a scientifically designed medical detox from sugar and all carb foods that turn to sugar. You simply take out the bad crap and replace it with good foods...plenty of good foods. There's a good reason why I call this the *The Method Approach: 14 Day Slimdown.*

Are you still not convinced you to need to pencil in a detox on your calendar for the next 14 days?

When a person consumes sugar, the tongues taste receptors are activated. Then, signals are sent to the brain, lighting up reward pathways and causing a surge of feel-good hormones, like dopamine, to be released. Sugar "hijacks the brain's reward pathway," explained neuroscientist Jordan Gaines. And while stimulating the brain's reward system with a piece of chocolate now and then is pleasurable and harmless, when the reward system is activated too much, then we start to run into problems.

There is really only one logical thing to do to start the journey of kicking the habit, and that is with a detox.

Here are my prescriptions for detecting the signs you need to detox.

Find out more about the program online at www.coachsyl.com. You can also scan the QR Code for quick access. 

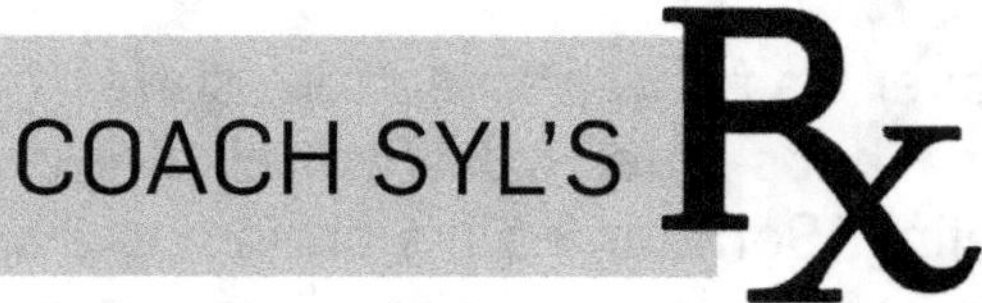

FLF DISORDER: FEEL LIKE FLUFF

You wake up feeling crappy. Your energy is low, and joy is replaced by despair. Even if you are thin and have toxic symptoms, a detox can help heal you quickly. The systems can include, fatigue, brain fog, achiness, digestive problem, allergy, and headache.

Most of us don't associate what we're eating with how we

feel. With my 14-day "Slimdown Detox" plan you will learn how to combat this needless suffering and feel good again in just a few days.

You Can't Lose Weight and Keep it Off?

The scientific establishment sells the message that losing weight is just a matter of calories in - calories out and about eating less and exercising more. How's that working out for you? Probably not so well!

The problem is, the scientific establishment is either unaware or doesn't care about the established science. Science says sugar and flour calories are very different from all the other foods.

First, they trigger addiction and overeating. Second, the combo spikes insulin production and inflammation occurs. This, in turn, makes you store belly fat and blocks your ability to feel full; a double whammy guaranteed to mess up any attempt at long-term weight loss. Case closed:

You can't Control Sugar and Carb Cravings (Think Food Addiction)

Sugar and wheat flour are biologically addictive. The science behind it is conclusive. Yet, we are quick to blame the fat person for being a lazy glutton. Imagine the fat person's feelings of shame and guilt.

Truth be told, it's not your fault. The food industry has hijacked your biology. It has executed a hostile takeover of your taste buds, brain chemistry, hormones, and metabolism.

Over 300 food industry insiders spilled the beans to Michael Moss in his book, *Salt, Sugar, and Fat*. Moss explains that the food industry hires "craving experts" to create the "bliss point" of junk food for purposes of creating "heavy users" and increase their "stomach share."

Sugar is the new nicotine. It's eight times more addictive than cocaine. If you depend on willpower to lose weight, you will fail. You need to use science to unhook yourself from the addictive power of sugar, wheat flour and hyper-palatable, hyper-processed, food-like substances (or "non-food junk" as Dr. Aviva Romm calls it).

YOU HAVE NEVER DETOXED

Most of us have never consumed delicious, wholesome, toxin-free food for 14 days in a row. At the end of a two-week detox, you will realize that your normal state is not your optimal state. Think of it as a two-week tune-up, a super-quick, super-easy way to supercharge your health.

YOU NEED A STAY-CATION

All of us stray from healthy living; too little sleep, too little exercise, too much bad food, excess stress, and not enough personal time.

The best way to reset your life is with a 14-day detox, and a good detox will have the following.

- Simple, delicious foods
- No toxins or drugs (sugar, flour, processed foods, trans fats or alcohol)
- Self-nurturing practices; deep breathing, sleeping 7-8 hours a night
- Moderate exercise
- Increased vitality

All this resets your body and mind back to their original factory settings—quickly!

PROGRESS NOTES

"Detox" refers to removing toxins from the body.

Sugar is the cause of more deaths every year than Cocaine and Heroin combined

Think about how you feel. Do you have:

- Low Energy
- Fatigue
- Allergies
- Aches
- Headaches

These can be signs of sugar addiction

Reset your body chemistry with a 14-Day Detox

- Simple foods
- No sugar
- No drugs or alcohol
- Plenty of rest; deep breathing
- Moderate exercise

Sylvia Williams

"DROP THE GYM" PRESCRIPTION

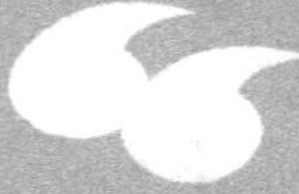

"Physical fitness is not only one of the most important keys to a healthy body, but it is also the basis of dynamic and creative intellectual activity."

John F. Kennedy

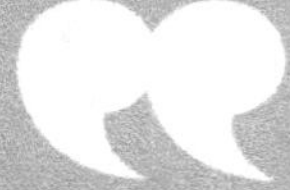

Sylvia Williams

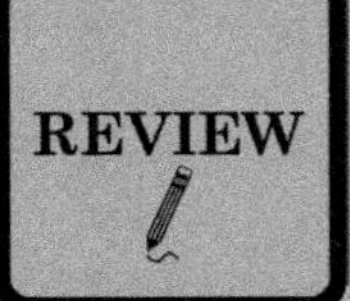

"10 years ago, after having my final child ,I went to Weight Watchers, and it worked! Then the weight came back, so I went back, and so the story goes.... it was a yo-yo, until one day it no longer worked!

My husband would always say to me, if you want to lose it, you gotta move it! Those were words I did NOT want to hear! I detested running or working out. I was the perfect member of the gym! They got my money but not my time!

Then menapause hit, Weight Watchers not only stopped working, but the reverse began happening. I felt that I could see my waistline increasing daily. My next move was a doctor visit. I hoped that the blood tests would reveal the cause of the weight increase.

I remember talking to Syl. She told me that losing 20 pounds, was totally obtainable. I didn't believe her. I think I said something like, 'If you can help me drop 20 pounds, I'll kiss your feet! It looks like I've got some feet to kiss because here I am....MORE than 20 pounds of fat, gone! Not only did I lose the weight, but I'm also committed to this NEW LIFE!"

—Client

Do I have to spend hours in the gym?

The simple answer is, no, you do not have to spend hours in the gym. In fact, spending hours in the gym may not help you at all if your eating habits are unhealthy and your vision of why you are on this journey is unclear.

Of course, I don't mean that the gym is a bad idea. It can be a great idea. But if you are looking for a simple cure for bad habits, then the gym isn't going to work.

Ask anyone from your doctor to your hairdresser how to lose weight, and you will hear some variation of the four timeless words: "Eat less, move more." But exactly how long do you need to work out to lose weight?

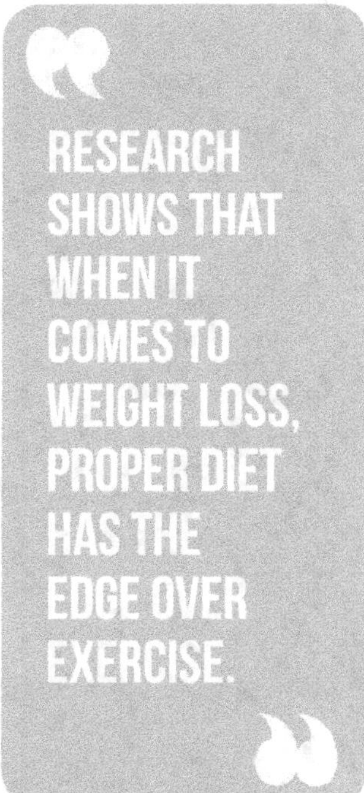

On the surface, it's good advice: losing weight is about creating an energy (calorie) deficit. Simple math reveals that when you burn more calories than you take in, your body pulls fuel from somewhere else - your fat stores.

But, how much exercise is needed to lose weight? Are there specific weight-loss workouts that help you reach your goals?

If you're fired up from the frustration of past weight loss failures, you may be tempted to try to burn more calories by cranking out more miles on the treadmill or doing double-sessions of spinning classes and yoga.

You might even try the latest wheat-germ-and-broccoli / no-butter-after-3-oclock p.m. / coffee-in-your-mutton-stew diet!

However, extreme fitness routines and extreme dieting aren't the answer. The real answer is much more common sense.

For most people, though, "eat less, move more" isn't practical advice. It's easier to say than to do. It's true, but so what? If you followed the advice, you'd end up a despondent, hungry jogger. Probably not what you're aiming for.

Research shows that when it comes to weight loss, proper diet has the edge over exercise. But, of course, people who combine diet and exercise lose more weight, faster.

Not all exercise is created equal. Some forms burn more calories than others. Contrary to popular belief, you don't have to sweat for hours a day to see results. Just 120 minutes of moderate intensity exercise a week can start to shrink your waistline, according to the American College of Sports Medicine.

I like to say 4 days a week for 30 minutes will keep the doctor and the fat away! Exercising more can accelerate your fat loss, as long as you follow a few simple guidelines.

If it's been a while since you've exercised, any type of physical activity will be new, so it not important what you do for the first several weeks. Simply doing something instead of nothing is beneficial. Walk, hike, cycle, jog, row, dance, swim, repeat.

In the beginning, your priority should be to establish the exercise habit. For that, shorter, more frequent workouts are best.

Here is my prescription to learn to exercise the right way.

Tired of failed diets and training programs? Checkout how much change is possible with The Method Approach. Scan the QR Code for quick access.

COACH SYL'S ℞

The right way combines the fundamentals of resistance training with higher intensity cross-training and incorporates all the elements of movement required for human survival.

These workouts produce strength and energy. They are fun and diverse, and, believe it or not, just like other cell nutrient requirements, you will come to crave rather than dread them!

You will become stronger, leaner and fitter quicker. Moreover, you will not develop disproportional muscle size; you will not incur repetitive strain injuries, and you will never be bored to tears like at a typical gym.

Doing more and eating less is a hard way to stay lean and get healthy!

The human body is a complex system. It is a miraculous organism that requires a particular balance of foods (fuel) and careful handling for optimum performance.

When we eat food and move, a complex neurological and hormonal system is launched. Firing neurons change hormone production and ultimately determines if you are going to store fat, have high levels of systemic inflammation, develop a chronic disease or live a long and healthy life.

Even though most trainers still promote doing more and eating less, the quality of exercise and foods plays a far more important role than quantity.

Many studies suggest this, adding proof that hours of conventional exercise per week are unnecessary.

Even day-to-day cardiovascular benefits, like walking up a few flights of stairs without getting puffed, are achieved faster following high-intensity exercise compared to sustained longer duration exercise.

Short bursts of intense exercise workouts increase aerobic (cardiovascular) activity more effectively than extended moderate intensity exercise, suggesting that the intense exercise produce greater cardioprotective benefits!

HOW IT WORKS

Our digestive system, muscle tissue, fat tissue and hormonal system constantly communicate with our brain and nervous system. As long as the nervous system is 'fully connected' and you are fuelling and moving properly, your innate genetic intelligence ensures that your health and physique will take care of itself.

Your muscles and liver store sugar (known as glycogen) due to an evolutionary self-preservation mechanism. Because sugar burns faster than any other fuel, it is important that your body has easy access to the 'sugar stash' to quickly supply your system with the fuel needed to effectively hot-foot it out ofa a sticky situation.

When you start to move in a 'survival' mode, your nervous system detects this stimulus. Then, via a cascade of signals, it quickly tells your muscles to use up the stored glycogen.

If you do not do any exercise, those glycogen stores hardly

get used, and there are devastating consequences. There has never been a Type II diabetic, obese, cancer-ridden, heart-diseased wild human that lived a genetically congruent lifestyle away from civilization.

Translation: Primitive people do not become obese, or develop diabetes, cancer or heart disease. Remember, when embracing integrated modalities you are matching your lifestyle choices to your genetic requirements,

Sure, important anabolic hormones such as testosterone, GH, and IGF-1 will flood the system with "old school" bodybuilding style workouts too – it is just far less efficient and far more stressful on the body.

Because these workouts are brief but intense, a large stress response is activated during the time of the workout but will remain present only for a small amount of time, post workout.

When comparing this to pumping iron for hours and hours per week, the shorter more intense workout allows for greater anabolic recovery time to rebuild muscle tissue, create more blood vessels and gain more health benefits from the workout.

Don't worry ladies; because you naturally produce less testosterone than men, training the right way will not cause the growth of facial hair or any other masculine features. You will just become stronger, more toned and leaner, the way nature intended.

PROGRESS NOTES

The role of a gym in fitness and health is changing. Those long, hard, sweaty aerobic workouts have been shown to be unnecessary.

Exercise the right way

- Combine resistance with high-intensity cross training

- Quality of exercise and food is more important than quantity

- Short bursts of intense workouts increase aerobic activity more than conventional workouts

- As long as the nervous system is fully connected your DNA will ensure proper health

Remember: primitive people do not become obese, develop diabetes, cancer or heart disease.

Sylvia Williams

CHAPTER
5

TWO'S COMPANY PRESCRIPTION

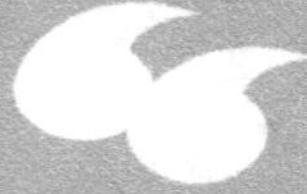

"One of the greatest enemies to achieving a total life makeover is the refusal to take responsibility for your own actions."

Robb Thompson

Sylvia Williams

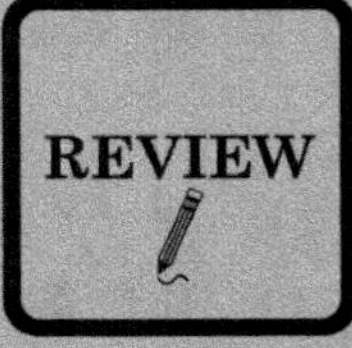

"I have struggled with my weight since the age of seven. I've tried all types of diets/programs. My most successful program was Weight Watchers, over 10 years ago, where I lost 40lbs, going from a size 22/24 to 14/16. However, 3 years later, I gained all 40lbs back, plus some.

I rejoined Weight Watchers many more times since, but never losing more than 10lbs. Just before turning 40, my weight would fluctuate between 210/215lbs, no matter what I ate, however after turning 40, my weight increased, and no matter what I did to lose, I continued to gain, finally hitting 250lbs. Did I mention, I'm only 5'2"?

Finally getting serious about this weight issue, I included it in my prayers. I'm excited to say my prayer was answered.

The difference between then and now is that I have a coach on this journey. Coach Syl, as the cliché goes, has been here and done that. Coach Syl has the wisdom & the knowledge along with the passion that makes this program so successful. On top of all of that, it is the accountability that she provides that helps keep me on track."

—Client

Does eating with others reduce overeating?

Will eating in the company of others help reduce overeating?

Two's company and three is never a crowd with this weight loss prescription. This phrase sums up the foundation of my saving grace during my own weight loss journey: **Don't eat alone.**

At the beginning of my journey, each meal eaten alone was like opening Pandora's box and discovering a black hole.

Needless to say, I was just a tad tempted to steer off my eating plan when I thought no one was watching; there were times I did just that. Although I wouldn't describe it as steering off the path, it was more like driving 80 mph on a narrow mountain road and then suddenly slamming my breaks to avoid toppling over the side of the mountain but realizing I was a little too late for that. It was pretty bad.

You know you've fallen off the proverbial weight loss wagon when you have to scarf down the burger and shake you got from the drive-through in the seven minutes it takes to get home to your family.

On the bright side, I didn't have many of those escapades. Otherwise, I'm not so sure I would have a transformation story to tell. I did, however, realize that when my husband or any person was around, I would inexplicably become much more disciplined in my eating. Go figure!

Seriously, there is power in NOT eating alone. In fact, there are several things you should not do alone.

Eating popcorn. The container holds enough popcorn for everyone in the theater and required one whole cow for the butter. Total calories? You don't want to know.

Shop for glasses. You're shopping for glasses because your vision sucks, so guess what frames the slick salesperson will try to dump off on you. All the ones that haven't sold since the store first opened.

Oh, and you should absolutely never try to play Monopoly or get on a seesaw alone.

I hope I've made the case that having others around when you're chowing down can and will have a significantly positive impact.

During the period when I went from a size 12 to a size 4 and had to decide what and how much I should eat, I came face-to-face with the beast all dieters dread; the relapse monster. It's a reality we all have to face off with at some point; can I maintain my results.

However, my golden ticket, the one I swear by till this day is to 'eat publicly.' This simply means most of my meals are around other people; some that I know and others I don't. The key is to not eat in a place where I can secretly indulge in the things that got me to my unhappy place, to begin with, but rather in a place that unintentionally holds me accountable to stay within the confines of my new healthy lifestyle. This place usually includes other people.

I'm sure you've noticed an uptick in solo diners at restaurants these days, and that you and your friends eat a lot of meals and snacks on your own? Thanks to our uber-busy lifestyles and that more people live alone than ever before (a record 27 percent of all households consist of one person), solo dining is the latest food trend.

A study done by the European Prospective Investigation of Cancer (EPIC Norfolk) that was started in 1993, followed 25,000 people between the ages of 40 and 80 over the past 20 years.

Researchers looked at how lifestyle and diet affect the onset of chronic diseases including diabetes and cancer. They discovered that

- Older single adults ate 2.3 fewer vegetable servings per day,

- Widows or widowers living alone consumed 1.1 fewer servings of vegetables per day than their married or cohabiting counterparts,

- Widows and widowers living with someone ate the same amount of vegetables as married or cohabiting people, highlighting the importance of social interaction.

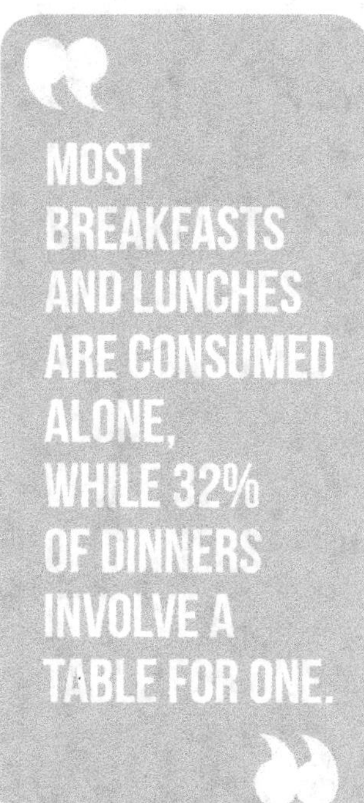

People's diet changes over time. Furthermore, eating healthy is influenced by a person's social environment, including factors like marriage, cohabitation, friendships and general social interacting. As people age, their diets become less balanced, and "… when older people are living alone their diet often suffers," says social epidemiology researcher, Annalijn Conklin.

A report from the NPD Group, a market research company, found that 55 percent of snacks and meals are eaten alone. Most breakfasts and lunches are consumed alone, while 32% of dinners involve a table for one.

Eating solo should be just as enjoyable and satisfying as a meal with friends or a partner. However, it often isn't. When you eat alone, you usually don't cook meals or choose healthy options. Leslie Heinberg, Ph.D., The Director of Behavioral Services at the Bariatric and Metabolic Institute at the Cleveland Clinic Foundation reports that "You often eat while doing other things, and that prevents you from picking up on hunger and satiety cues, which increases the likelihood of weight gain."

Keep these waistline-expanding traps in mind when you find yourself dining alone.

Dining at your Dashboard

It doesn't feel right to set a just one place at a table. Eating alone is a drag, and it leads a lot of people to head for the fast food joint and eat in their car. This makes you more prone to picking up high-calorie and less-healthy food, as well as to eating mindlessly. The result is in you not feeling "full" and overeating.

When you are in the company of others, you take your focus off of yourself and hopefully give someone else your undivided attention thus taking your mind off of eating, weight loss and yes the scale.

This prescription gives you the reasons to eat with others that may not seem like they have any connection to weight loss.

Want to start eating healthier? Get diet and recipe advice on our website. Scan the QR Code for quick access.

COACH SYL'S ℞

1. Eating with others allows you to be present

Technology can do wonders for your life, but it can also distract you from being fully present, especially around the dining table. When you constantly check your email, look up the latest shopping deal, or log into social media to see what's happening with your friends' you're robbing yourself of important time to be aware of your needs.

Eating at a table with others is great, providing there are no distractions, like smartphones. Notice when you are with a group of friends how many of them are not really there. They are in the cyber world. It would be funny if it weren't so tragic.

Take charge and get everyone at the table to turn off their phones during dinner, if you can. Use the opportunity to savor food flavors, and listen. Recognize when you're full and stop eating.

2. Eating with others is a networking tool

Having a lunch buddy can foster some in-house networking with colleagues. It can also help maintain friendly relationships with your professional peers and make connections to colleagues in distant departments "Left up to our own devices, we end up having lunch with people who are on the same teams as us," says Michael Soto, co-founder of Spark Collaboration, which introduces co-workers for one-on-one meetings to help build relationships. "We encourage people to reach out and talk to people from different social circles."

Eating, or just having coffee with someone from another

department is an important approach to breaking down the silos that exist in many organizations.

Some employers encourage this inter- and intra-office unity with organized lunches, brown bag workshops, and other sponsored events. It's cheap, and it satisfies the all-important biological necessity: Everyone has to eat.

3. *Eating with others makes you happier*

"If we can foster an environment where people are establishing friendships with the people around them, people will be happier at their job, almost regardless of the work they're doing," says Andrew Horn, co-founder and CEO of Tribute, a video-montage platform, and frequent speaker on networking and communication.

Eating with an office friend can lessen the dread of trudging to work every day. Lunch buddies have a few minutes to kick back, discuss solutions to to work related problems or simply shoot the breeze.

Says Horn: "Even if it's not the most natural thing for you to go and spend time with your co-workers, spending the time to develop those relationships is something I think you'll be proud of as a human being and a professional in the long run."

BUT if you absolutely have to eat alone be sure to watch out for these things:

Portion size

Often cans or jars of food are meant for four people. This means the nutrition information on the container will be per quarter of the jar. If you're preparing a dinner for one, it's tempting to throw half of the sauce in without thinking. This usually results in eating double the recommended amount.

Similarly, other things like zoodles and cauliflower rice can be hard to measure out, so consider referring to cup size.

If you do prepare a large amount in at one time, have some Tupperware on hand and dish things into freeze-able portions. This prevents you from eating the same thing for several days in a row.

Quick-fix food

When you make a meal for yourself, you are less likely to put in as much work as when you cook for family or friends. That doesn't mean, however, that you have to rely on convenience food like takeaways or microwave dishes. Metabolizing whole foods uses about 50 percent more calories than processed. Another benefit is eating fresh is often tastier and will leave you fuller and with more energy. You don't have to create a gourmet feast. Just throw some meat on the grill with plenty of fresh vegetables instead of relying on a ready meal.

Distractions

Eating alone isn't entertaining, so you'll probably find your-self doing other things at the same time, such as watching TV, catching up on work or checking social media. This means you might not be as on top of what you're actually consuming - which could lead to overeating.

When you eat a full meal alone, take advantage of the alone time to concentrate on yourself. It might seem awkward at first but focus on enjoying your food rather than getting rid of the hunger feeling. You will appreciate the flavors a lot more than if you are alone. If it's just a quick snack eaten on the sofa, don't take the whole bag/box/tub. Dish out a manage-able portion and put the rest away.

Speedy Eating

Like eating while distracted, when you are alone you're also more likely to consume everything too fast. When dining with others, you take more time to savor the moment, but solo snacking is a different matter. If you eat without thinking, you're less likely to be aware of when you're actually full. Take time with your meals and see them as more than just a necessity - food is meant to be enjoyed. You bet your bottom it is!

PROGRESS NOTES

Plan to eat with others to reduce overeating. Additional benefits include being more engaged in the moment, networking with co-workers and being happier.

If you do eat alone, follow these tips: If you do eat alone, follow these tips:

- Be aware of portion size

- Try not to be distracted by social media or work. Savor the moment, just as you would with a group of friends

- Eat fresh food, not fast food.

- Cook for yourself just as you would for others; be prepared to freeze the extras for later.

CHAPTER 6

NO MORE "FAT CLOTHES" COVER-UP PRESCRIPTION

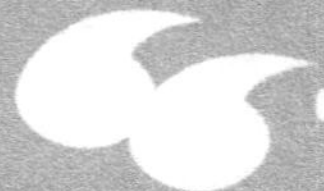

"A wise man should consider that health is the greatest of human blessings, and learn how, by his own thought, to derive benefit from his illnesses."

Hippocrates

Sylvia Williams

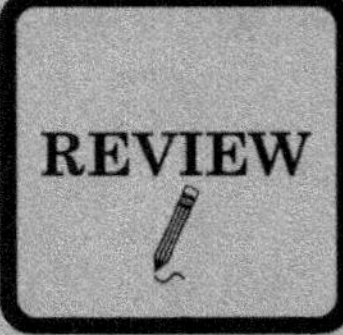

"I am so grateful for the journey I have been on to improve my health. I was blown away by my before and after picture, and I was blown away by what we have accomplished in a short amount of time: 60 pounds and counting...Whoa! I literally prayed for help, and God answered. Every day He has strengthened me to tap into His power to change.

I thank God for my hubby, Apostle Deon Hunt, and my little peeps hanging in there with me on the no processed foods and clean eating change and for encouraging me. "Momma, you are not supposed to be eating that, put it down!!" I encourage everyone facing a challenge to ask God for help and listen for the answer. God is always faithful!! He gives us strength and then we have to use it wisely.

Taking every step in the right direction matters. The journey of one thousand miles literally begins with a single step. Keep taking steps, no matter how small they may seem, until you reach the goal. You will look up and be amazed at how far you have come."

—Client

Can wearing "FAT CLOTHES" cause me to gain weight?

No, only eating too much sugar and/or carbs will cause you to gain weight. Wearing baggy clothes just won't remind you of your weight like tighter fitting work clothes will.

Gone are the days, it seems, when standard professional attire was a nicely tailored skirt and blouse. And, even if nicer clothes are a requirement, it is easy now to find a nice dress of knit fabric that fits like a baggy sweater.

Casual wear is no different. Where we once might have worn jeans of stiff, unforgiving denim, most jeans today are made of a blend that allows them to stretch.

It's like the yoga pant epidemic. You can go to any mall in America and surely you will find a slew of women dressed as if they're on their way to the local Planet Fitness, only to discover they haven't seen the inside of a gym since high school. This has become the new fashion statement with companies popping up like Lululemon and Fabletics with their fashionable elastic attire that's designed for most occasions. And we have definitely been drinking that Kool-Aid; myself included.

It seems that instead of keeping our waistlines in line with our wardrobes, we have wardrobes of clothes that expand as we do. I'm not suggesting that stretchy clothing causes a person to gain weight any more than muumuus do, but it doesn't help the cause.

Just think back to the days of wearing Jordache or Sergio Valente jeans. Talk about unforgiving brands. I swear if you gained one ounce, trying to get the zipper up was the equivalent of doing one of Shawn T-s workout videos. You had to lie flat on the bed and squirm like a wounded worm to even button them up.

Now we've gone from stiff denim to pants made of rayon and lycra spandex. These pants might as well have a notice in the pockets saying, "No worries, we've got your back(side). You can gain up to 20 pounds before you have to buy a larger size.

Case closed. Eating too much sugar and/or carbs causes weight gain. Wearing baggy clothes, on the other hand, just won't remind you of your weight like tighter fitting work clothes will.

Speaking of the tighter-fitting clothes, consider buying a smashing outfit you'd love to have in your goal size. It's almost like telling a child she can have cookies once she finishes her homework. Motivation can be found in many things and ways. In this scenario you're telling yourself you could look hot or cute in that fabulous new dress or designer skinny jeans when you lose enough weight to fit into them. This could give you the extra push to pass on dessert or second helpings of dinner. It could also give you the extra drive to go to the gym or run an extra 20 minutes. Any motivation is always welcomed during a weight loss journey, even something as simple as clothing.

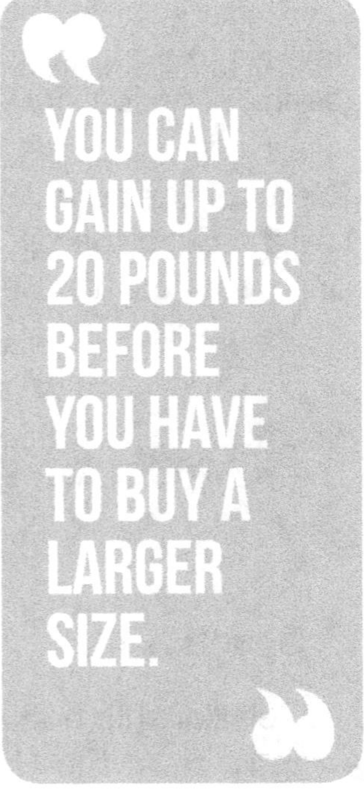

My item of choice was a pair of Guess jeans my husband bought me from an outlet store. At the time, I could only get the jeans to my knees. Needless to say, they were too small. However, I held on to them during my weight loss journey, and I would try them on every three to four weeks, and one day I slipped them right on.

My item of choice was a pair of Guess jeans my husband This may not sound groundbreaking, but you have to understand, I had these jeans for well over 5 years. They even had the tags on them, but you know what was funny, once I was finally able to wear them I realized I didn't even like the style. They had a weird bell-bottom cut, so I ended up giving them away, but the satisfaction I felt knowing that I did the work to transform my body to the point I was able to fit in a clothing item that was collecting dust was the biggest confidence boost ever. I felt in control.

Here is my prescription for identifying non-food weight gaining contributors you may be suffering from.

Discover the actual reasons why you're gaining weight. Scan the QR Code for quick access to our website with useful resources.

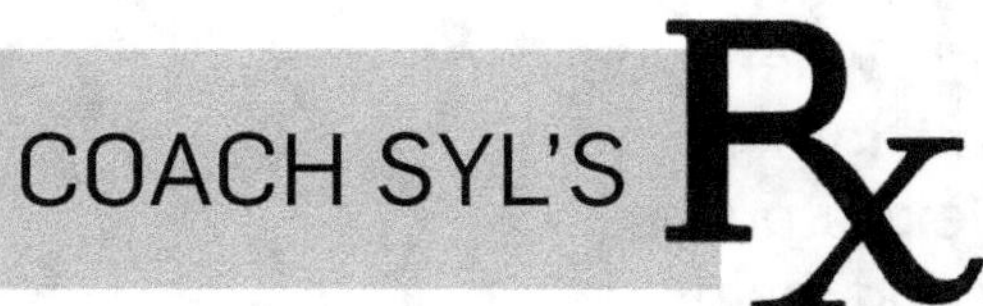

1. Genetics

The relationship between obesity and genetics is well known. A report from the University of Sussex found that the children of obese parents are 35% to 45% more likely to become obese than children of average weight parents.

Genetic obesity is not totally predetermined, it's more of a predisposition. The messages our brain sends to our genes can have a significant effect on which obesity genes are expressed and the ones that are not.

Third-world cultures rapidly develop obesity when they begin eating typical Western world diet. Their genes didn't change, the signals sent to their genes changed.

Science has established that there are genetic components that affect our vulnerability to gain weight. Studies on identical twins demonstrate this, including a finding published in the New England Journal of Medicine N Engl J Med. 1990 May 24.

2. Food Addiction

The Journal of Neuroscience, Volume 134, Issue 3, 2005 reports that highly engineered junk foods cause potent stimulation of the reward centers in our brains.

Guess what else does? Drugs like cocaine, alcohol, nicotine, and cannabis.

Moreover, junk foods can cause full-scale addiction in vulnerable individuals. The addicts lose control over their eating, in exactly the same way as alcoholics lose control over their drinking.

3. Insulin

Insulin is a vital hormone that regulates energy storage, among other things. Insulin tells fat cells to store fat and to hold on to the existing fat.

The Western diet causes insulin resistance in many cultures. This elevates insulin levels throughout the body, causing energy to be stored in fat cells instead of being available for use.

4. Certain Medications

Many pharmaceutical drugs can cause weight gain as a side effect. Examples include diabetes medication, antidepressants, antipsychotics, etc.

These drugs don't cause a "willpower deficiency," instead, they alter the function of the body and brain, making the body store fat instead of burning it.

5. Leptin

A hormone that is critical in obesity is Leptin. This hormone is produced by fat cells. Its role is to send signals to the hypothalamus (the part of the brain that regulates food intake) that we're full and need to stop eating.

Obese people have lots of fat and leptin. The problem is that the leptin isn't working as it should because for some reason the brain becomes resistant to it.

This is called leptin resistance and considered to be a leading factor in the development of obesity.

6. Misinformation

People all over the world are misinformed about health and nutrition. I think the main reason is that food companies sponsor scientists and major health organizations all around the world.

For example, the Academy of Nutrition and Dietetics (the largest organization of nutrition professionals in the world) is heavily sponsored by companies such as Coca-Cola, Kellogg's and Pepsico.

The American Diabetes Association is sponsored by drug

companies making millions of dollars per year, companies that directly profit from the failed low-fat advice.

Even the official guidelines promoted by the government seem to be designed to protect the interests of the corporations instead of encouraging the health of individuals.

How can people make the right choices if they're constantly being lied to by the government, health organizations and the professionals that are supposed to know what to do?

The point of this chapter is to open people's minds to the fact that something other than "individual responsibility" may be the cause of the obesity epidemic.

The way our foods and society have been engineered are all important factors that must be corrected if we are to reverse this problem on a global scale.

PROGRESS NOTES

Loose, baggy clothes won't make you gain weight, but they can make you less aware of the weight you are gaining.

To help you stay on track, try at least sometimes to wear clothes that won't fit properly if you gain weight.

It can even help to have "goal" pants or dresses... nice things that you can slide into once you lose those extra pounds!

CHAPTER 7

TATTLE-TALE PRESCRIPTION

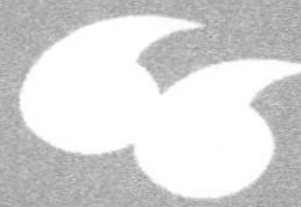

"Don't sacrifice yourself too much, because if you sacrifice too much there's nothing else you can give and nobody will care for you"

Karl Lagerfeld

Sylvia Williams

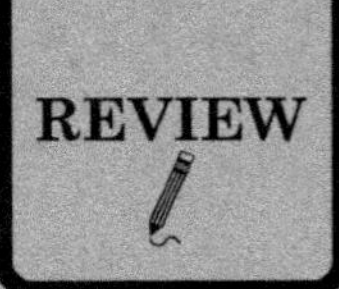

"I had an epiphany one night while shopping for a new dress. I didn't like the way I looked, and I knew that I needed to change my ways. So I went home and looked into the program.

I knew a little bit about it because my friend had previously joined and was very successful with an 80-pound weight loss. When I signed up, I was committed, and because of that commitment, I reaped the rewards. The rewards included short workouts, uncomplicated nutrition, and accountability.

The nutrition knowledge is another huge component and is what saved me during a tough time. I was off of work for 3 months due to a car accident, and I was devastated. Although the weight was coming off, I was scared it was going to come back because I wasn't working out.

Coach Syl gave me the much-needed support and guidance I needed. So while I couldn't work out, I continued to follow her nutrition guidance and totally changed my eating habits. Because of that, I was able to reach my goal. I'm down 60 pounds! She saved me both emotionally and physically!!"

—Client

Will telling friends and colleagues about my weight loss journey help me stay committed?

The jury is out. What will help is showing results.

I remember when I made a conscious decision to publicly share my journey, with not only my clients but with my Facebook friends and their friends, etc. It was a liberating feeling. I wasn't concerned with how I appeared; I was more interested in the accountability I could gain from putting myself out there publicly.

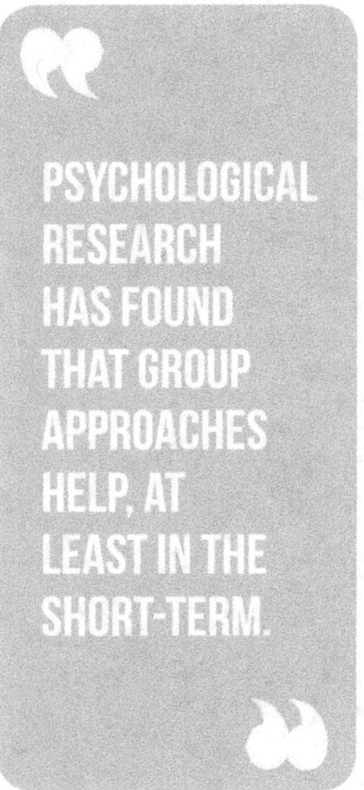

At first, it was awkward, trying to figure out what I should and shouldn't share and if some things were TMI. I also, wondered if people would tire of my sharing, or think I was showing off. But in the end, I realized maybe all of the above were true, but the truth I chose to glean from my experience was that the reward for sharing was bigger than the sacrifice.

Every post and share was proof of the commitment I had made to this form of accountability. I knew that I couldn't allow myself to be caught doing the opposite of what I was sharing or shame on me. It probably was one of the single most impactful things I did on my journey after discovering my Why.

Unbeknownst to me, in my pursuit of accountability via social media, I discovered I had become a luminary for many women and men. This further confirmed the not set out to become, but by opening my journey to others, was elected to be.

Statistically, if you expand your announcement to greater

numbers of people than just your closest circle, the greater the reinforcement you have to stay committed.

Public announcements of plans, any plans, have built-in reinforcement value. The core feature of the very successful Weight-Watchers program is the meetings of dieters sharing their goals and achievements with one another.

Psychological research has found that group approaches help, at least in the short-term.

A recent study by a psychology professor at Dominican University discovered that more than 70% of 267 participants who sent weekly progress reports to a friend reported successful goal achievement, compared to only 35% of those who kept their goals to themselves.

It's easier to stay on a weight loss plan when you have support, check in for accountability and have an exercise buddy.

The following are my prescriptions for finding support.

Join a like-minded group and achieve results together. Find out more on our website. Scan the QR Code for quick access.

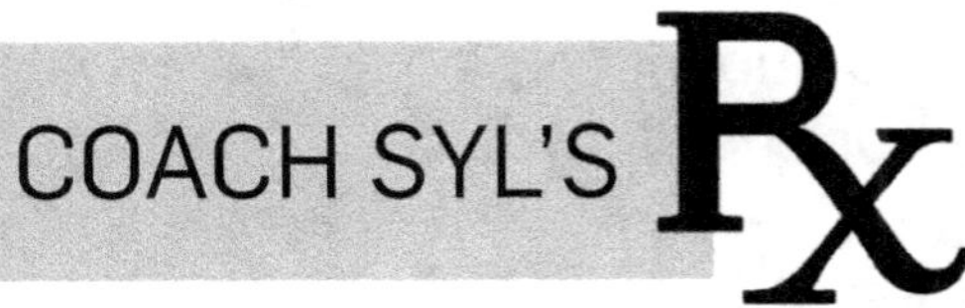

COACH SYL'S ℞

Join a weight loss program:

A weight loss program that includes group support, discussions about exercise and diet and accountability, is a good option.

In one study, participants who enrolled in a weight-loss program with friends kept weight off longer than programs without friends. In addition to teaming up with friends, the study enrollees were given not just standard treatment, but also social support. Two-thirds of those who joined with friends had kept their weight off six months after the meetings ended. In contrast, only a quarter of those who attended solo had achieved that same success.

Showing versus just telling someone about your weight loss appears to have remarkable success.

Strong social circles are seen as very effective in combatting obesity. In a 2013 research study published in Translational Behavioral Medicine, participants who published their weight loss progress on Twitter lost more weight than those who kept their progress to themselves.

A publicized task allows people to push you the advice and motivation you need before you have to search for a solution.

Commit to the benefits of public goal setting:

There is something about common topic public announcements that motivates readers to respond. If, when you tell colleagues or customers about your diet plans, you hand them your business card containing your personal email address, be prepared to receive a great deal of positive feedback. Moreover, I have a sense that your announced plans will motivate many of your contacts to get on the diet wagon.

Get Over Guilt for Public Failure:

It's harder to fail when you've got people pulling for you. The larger your audience, the greater the pressure on you to succeed. By the same token, those in your audience that provide feedback will feel the pressure for them to do the same.

Add More Accountability:

Guilt is a consequence of not being accountable for your actions. Therefore it's what drives people to accomplish their goals.

The downside of taking your weight loss journey independently is, being independent. When no one is looking over your shoulder, and you set your own goals and deadlines, things can go sideways rather quickly.

The trim little angel on one shoulder quietly whispers in your ear that task needs completing, but the loud fat devil on the other shoulder gets you to lose focus.

Telling people like your friends and colleagues about your diet plans can be a game changer.

So, go public with your weight loss plans, and when you see people, they will undoubtedly inquire about your progress. This will certainly keep you on your toes.

PROGRESS NOTES

Go public with your diet plans to get reinforcement from your circle of family, friends and colleagues.

To stay on plan, try these action items:

- Have support, from any source

- Use a structured program

- Use a program personalized for you

- Announce your goals on social media

- Show results [photos] vs. just telling

- Share progress reports

You will find that you are not making this journey alone, and maybe even that your story inspires others!

CHAPTER
8

THE CHALLENGE PRESCRIPTION

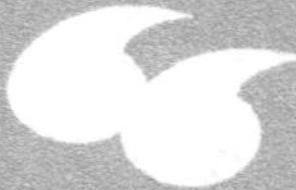

"It's better to be healthy alone than sick with someone else."

Phil McGraw

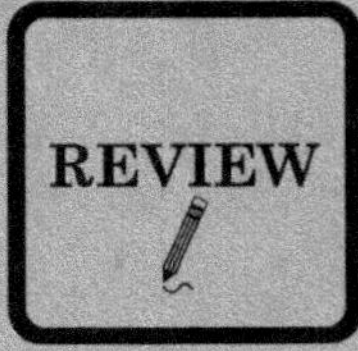

"This is the first time in a long time I feel strong. I have an immensely stressful timetable (it seems like we all do these days) so I have limited work out time. The 30- minute workouts are perfect. I have never sweated so much in my life. I've had a remarkable experience, so far, overcoming my insecurities and plowing through self-doubt."

—Client

Can short challenges help me lose weight?

Absolutely!

However, short-term diet challenge successes are usually short term as well. It sometimes takes longer to see improvements in fitness levels following short-term intense fitness plans when compared with long-term programs.

Specifically, researchers found that when a group of healthy women and men with similar fitness levels completed 24 high-intensity training sessions, those that participated a 3-week crash course showed no improvement in their fitness levels.

But, those that did the 24 workouts spread out over eight weeks showed significant improvement in their fitness levels.

In general, setting, and meeting goals (aka, challenges) can become a habit. There are bad habits, like eating too much of the wrong foods. Good habits are the ones that help make you a better person, i.e., stronger, faster, healthier.

A challenge can be viewed as a goal, i.e., I want to be a size 6 again. The steps you take to achieve a goal are called Objectives, which are measurable, i.e., 1. Consume no more than 1200 calories per day, 2. Eat nothing made from wheat flour. 3. Walk around the block six times every day.

A small percentage of people are goal-setting nuts, and an equally small percentage are goal-setting challenged. Most people, the classic 80%, fall somewhere in the middle.

Irrespective of where you are on that continuum a terrific tool for developing the short- or long-term challenge habit is a big To Do chart. Get a big Dry-Erase calendar board and create short challenges.

Multiple short challenges are terrific. A short challenge might be, "No wheat flour bread for seven days."

Build up the number of concurrent short challenges and don't make the challenges too tough. You just want to develop the "habit" of setting goals, and objectives. That habit will be an immense help in your development of the good health habits you seek.

When you complete a challenge, draw a line through it, and in a right column write a number value, like 10, for each completed challenge. If you fall short on a challenge, place a lesser number in the right-hand column.

One of the biggest trends in diet and fitness programs are short-term challenges. Do they work?

There are pros and cons to these challenges, and they are usually related to individual differences.

Beginning a diet challenge and integrating it into your lifestyle can be daunting. A short-term holistic weight loss challenge can seem a little less daunting if it is structured into a manageable time-frame.

Here is my prescription for considering the pros and cons of short challenges.

Scan the QR Code for proof that weight loss is both a short term and long-term goal/challenge worth taking up.

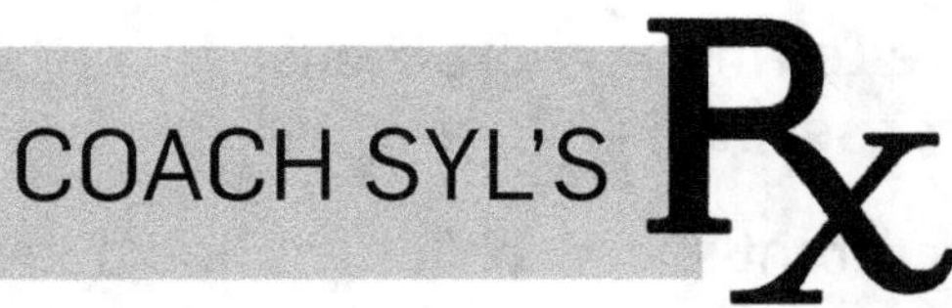

Pros

Starting a weight loss challenge often produces a surge of motivation which can hopefully be sustained well past the completion of the challenge.

Lead-in to Long-Term Strategies

A diet program done correctly should inspire you to make lasting changes to your lifestyle. "Slow and steady wins the long race."

A good program will educate you to make informed choices about the foods you eat, daily movement, and wellness.

Tap into Your Competitive Side

We all have a competitive drive. Fitness challenges are great for those that like a little friendly competition to get their juices flowing. It's important to remember that your toughest competitor is yourself.

Sense of Community

Diet program challenges are often done in groups. When you show up at a group meeting either virtual or in person, you're with people who know exactly what you are going through. The close bonds become a catalyst for action and an inspiration for victory.

Give You Goals

Short-term challenges can be set by your coach. A benefit of these challenges is that you receive clear direction. A good challenge allows you to identify a goal and set a time frame. The BEST weight loss program challenges are tailored to best fit the individual.

Cons

Some programs can encourage overtraining. This is a common shortcoming of short-term challenges. Anything that encourages atypical dieting or overtraining is not good physically or mentally.

You want these challenges to produce weight loss, more energy and build your strength and fitness.

Unrealistic Expectations

Before and after photos are inspiring, but don't forget every person's body is different. No two individuals will react to a specific program in the same way. Make sure that when you set a goal with your trainer that it is realistic and attainable.

Unbalanced

Balance is key! The most effective and sustainable training programs alternate heavy and light workout days. All training challenges should promote adequate rest and recovery to ensure participants aren't going to burn out.

Ends abruptly

Once you finish the challenge, you may be left thinking, 'What's next?' A successful challenge should always provide you with pathways to ongoing success and long-term health and fitness goals. Look for these pathways in the programs and the group you're training with.

If you need that extra little bit of motivation and structure to fire up your fitness regime, then short-term fitness challenges may be the thing for you! Before jumping into one, do your research, keep a healthy attitude and be realistic.

Also, reward yourself with something you looooove, other than food, if you reach your target number. See Chapter 10 for a list of super self-rewards.

PROGRESS NOTES

Do short-term challenges work?

Absolutely, but there are pros and cons. The key is finding challenges that work for you. Work with your coach to identify several short-term challenges.

- Make sure you clearly understand the goals for the challenge.

- Be sure to discuss whether the challenge is realistic.

- Share your goals with others in your fitness community.

- Organize a "friendly competition" to encourage yourself and your fitness friends to pursue your goals

- Plan how you will reward yourself for meeting a goal.

- Track your goals and whether you meet them on a white board.

Sylvia Williams

CHAPTER 9

ACCOUNTABILITY PRESCRIPTION

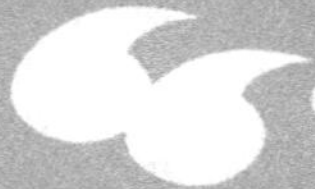

"Defeat doesn't finish a man, quit does. A man is not finished when he's defeated. He's finished when he quits."

Richard Nixon

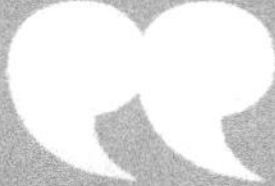

Sylvia Williams

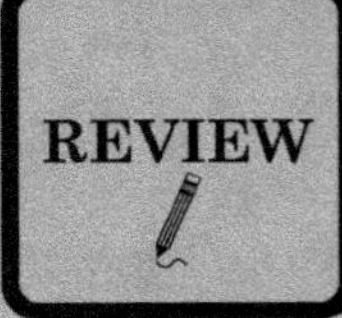

"Reality set in when my parents needed to be in an assisted/independent living home. I had been working with my dad, helping him get in and out of a wheelchair when my back and knees began yelling at me. I remember looking around the home at the patients with canes, walkers, and wheelchairs and noticing that most of the patients were overweight. At that moment I thought, "I do not want to be in that predicament when I'm that age," and I vowed it was time to do something about it.

I sensed that the epiphany came from God. I took action, and the support I have received is amazing. I used to wear a size 1x-2x in tops and size 16-18 in bottoms, and I now am in a size L in tops and 10-12 in bottoms! I am going to continue!"

—Client

How can Accountability help me lose weight?

Contrasted with responsibility, accountability involves liability or fault. When trying to lose or maintain weight loss, you need more than just willpower.

I've always said that you can give a person the exact formula for weight loss and chances are it still won't be enough. Most people gasp when I say that, but it's true. Knowing exactly what you need to eat and which workouts are best still leave many dieters scratching their head over disappointing results.

I bet you remember weight loss fitness programs you believed contained all the information you needed, but for some crazy reason, you still didn't reach your goal.

The likely reason involves accountability.

Without the proper type and amount of accountability, most people don't stick to a program long enough to see their desired outcome. In short, being held accountable is just as important as the program itself.

Just ask the Biggest Loser contestants who go home after the second or third week. Why is it that a significantly larger percentage of this group fall off the diet wagon than those that make it to the finals? They've been given all the tools they need to eat properly and workout, but they all were short of one element. Accountability. It's the secret sauce to any transformational success story, including my own.

A client of mine once said, "I never knew I could miss your accountability program so much." Others have told me that it is the one thing that the other programs they've been apart of either didn't have or didn't do well. Another client described having me as their coach as like having a Ford. You can always count on Ford.

I believe that if I'm going to have a program that helps

high-achieving women adopt a healthy lifestyle, I better put plenty of speed bumps on the road because this is what ultimately will help a person stay in line with their journey. Those speed bumps are check-in times, updates and goal setting.

Without too much psychobabble, people respond to the expectations of others and in this context, that comes in the form of having a coach who will hold you accountable.

It's not enough to have the right tools for reaching your weight-loss goals; just ask Oprah, Mariah Carey and Janet Jackson. I'm certain they can afford all the tools a girl needs, but without the right accountability sauce you'll end up on the yo-yo train just as they have.

A study done by the American A study done by the American Society of Training and Development found that people have a 65% chance of completing a goal when they commit to someone, and this number increases when the commitment is specific. That someone can be a friend, family member or co-worker. However, in most cases they are not the best fit to hold you accountable and keep you accountable.

> A STUDY DONE BY THE AMERICAN SOCIETY OF TRAINING AND DEVEOLOPMENT FOUND THAT PEOPLE HAVE A 65% CHANCE OF COMPLETING A GOAL WHEN THEY COMMIT TO SOMEONE.

I've seen people team up with siblings and neighbors on their weight loss journey. At first things are great, but then they get 'THE CALL'. You know the one where your workout buddy says I don't think I'm going to be able to make it to the gym today or I had something come up I'm going to need to cancel. This ultimately takes you on the journey of many missed workouts, piled high excuses and the inevitable fall from the wagon.

In great programs, there are typically four types of accountability. The first is accountability to yourself, then to a partner, a group and lastly the public.

Until now we've viewed accountability as a principle, but it should be viewed as a method.

Here are my prescriptions to hold yourself accountable until you find the right coach!

Work with an Accountability Coach and begin enjoying these benefits and so much more. 

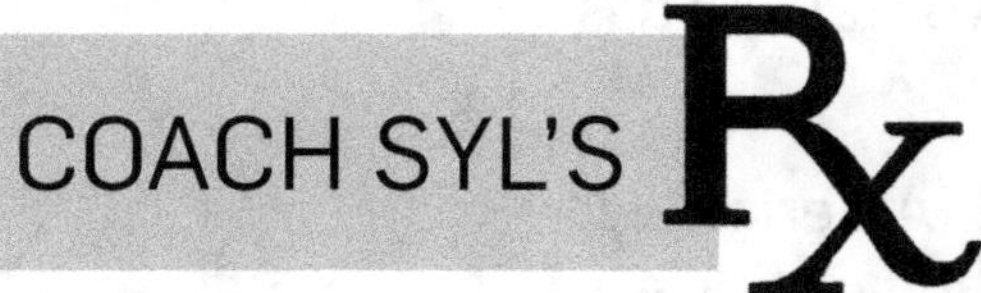

1. Bond with your Scale

You likely have a love-hate relationship with your scale. Scales are not a necessary tool, but it can be very helpful in your battle of the bulge. According to J. Graham Thomas, Ph.D., associate professor at the Miriam Hospital and Brown Medical Center in Providence, R.I., which operates the National Weight Control Registry.

Seventy-five percent of the 10,000 successful dieters enrolled in the Registry weigh weekly, and 38 percent weigh daily. They all learned to love the scale, particularly for monitoring weight-loss maintenance.

We all know weight is a nasty stealth creeper. The Registry

member uses the scale to identify creeping weight gain so they can take immediate corrective action.

2. Tape Measure

To determine weight loss or maintenance success use a cloth tape measure. When you measure your waistline, hips, bust, and even thighs and calves, you can record tangible progress toward your goal with detail that a scale can't provide. Because muscle takes up less volume than fat, you'll see inches drop, even when there might not be a corresponding change in weight. It's encouraging, and we need all the encouragement we can get.

3. Food Diary

Tracking with a food diary is an excellent tool and is easy to use. You can list calories, foods, or just mark an "X" on the calendar for every day you meet your daily goals.

A great accountability trick is writing down what you plan to eat before you eat it, not after. It increases your awareness and makes you think twice about food before you eat it.

4. Save Skinny Clothes

Some people keep a pair of "fat pants" in view as a reminder of what's in store if they fall off the wagon. Better, keep a pair of pants handy that you crave to fit into. Get rid of all fat clothes when you reach your goal, so you know that there's no going back."

5. Diet BFF

There are arguments for and against having a diet buddy. It seems like a good idea on its face, but there can be pitfalls; not losing weight pitfalls, but rather losing friends pitfalls. If you want to try partnering up with someone pick a Not Favorite Friend.

6. Make it Public

When only you know about **your weight-loss** plan and goals, it's easy to cheat. However, when you make the plan public, you'll feel a great deal more responsibility to meet your goals.

Tell your family the specifics of your goal, for example, how much weight you plan to lose by what date, or how many times per week you plan to exercise.

Post your goal to your social networking website of choice or keep a blog. Post pictures of **yourself** and share your success with friends and family members. They'll expect you to meet your goal, which will motivate you to honor your word.

7. Set your action goals

It's not enough to say you want to lose weight. Spell out the action goals that will make hitting your overall goals so easy! If you want to lose 15 pounds, how do you want to do it? One action goal might be:

"I will workout for 20 minutes three times/week."

Write down three action goals and look at them every day. Are you on top of your to-dos? If not, do what you need to get back on track and to end the week on a positive note.

To Me, from Me:

When you set a reminder alarm don't you find it hard to ignore it? What if you wrote yourself an actual email at night to yourself.

Only you will be reading it, but it can be incredibly motivating and helpful. Here's a sample of what you might write.

"Hi, Madison. I am so proud of the steps you are taking to change your body, life, and spirit. I am happy that you finally reached your threshold where enough is enough, and you've joined a program that will hold you accountable.

Diet wise, things went well today. The kale shake was amazing, and the lunch was delicious. You should feel good about yourself for eating lunch at the office instead of going out to eat. Tomorrow though, let's try to avoid eating those cookies that mom sent. I am also pumped over the workout that is on the schedule. Coach Syl is really kicking butt lately with workout plans. It's nice to not have to create them myself. I can't wait to 'feel the burn.'

See what I mean? How can you wake up, read that and not feel stoked for the day?

WHERE ARE YOU NOW?

Because you see yourself every day are you tuned in to the progress your body is making? Most likely not. And because of that, it's so easy to get frustrated and upset and just give up. Track your progress by knowing where you are right now.

Grab a camera and take a 'before' shot of you wearing just panties and a sports bra. Take your measurements (waist, thigh, hips, arm); and of course your weight (though this isn't the most ideal tracking element). Every two weeks repeat these tracking measurements so that you can compare and see proof-positive that your hard work is paying off!

SLOW CHANGES

Smart fitness professionals will tell you that diets don't work. Cutting back on your food or cutting out certain foods completely just won't cut it for losing weight. You'll just feel deprived and miserable. Cravings will erupt, your metabolism crash, and before you know it you've got your face in a bag of chips, grease on your hands and the weight you lost starts creeping back.

Instead of worrying about eating less, concern yourself with eating more of the healthy foods. Replace typical meals with healthier options. Make slow swaps in your diet. Love chips? Change to Pop Chips and stick to the right portions. Love lattes? Go for a latte that uses coconut milk with some stevia instead. Trust me, these small changes add up and can make a huge impact.

1.Stand Up for Yourself

One of the hardest challenges you face is dealing with others around you. They will complain about all the healthy foods, they will grumble about the interference of a new nutrition plan, and they will pressure you to "cheat for just one meal." Stand firm and ask them to support your efforts.

2.Contract with Yourself

Write your weight-loss plan in the form of a contract with yourself. Spell out the terms of your agreement by outlining your weight-loss plan. Include a summary of your goals and a complete description of how you will meet them.

For example, include your workout timetable and your diet plan. If your goal is to workout five days per week and only have one cheat day on the weekend, include that. Sign the document and post it where you will see it every day. If you feel yourself slipping back, reread the document and renew your agreement with yourself.

You will need support. Simply sitting down with your family and discussing your plans will make them feel involved and are more likely to support you and your goals.

3. Meal Plan Time

Every week, sit down with your favorite health-related cookbooks and tablet and plan out your week. Make your grocery list with your meal plan in mind and then stick to the list.

When you shop with a list, you are less likely to impulse buy, and you'll save money too. Then during the week, you know what you'll be eating, and you won't be tempted to make a stop to pick up food from the burger joint on the way home.

4. Go even if you don't Sweat

We all have days when we can't get in the mood to workout. But it's important, especially in the beginning, that you power through those times make fitness a habit and a part of your lifestyle.

On the days you just aren't feeling it, go anyway. If you go, you probably will stay because you took the time and went all that way and it would be silly to leave.

Let's face it, 90% of the time when you walk in you'll find some motivation and walk out feeling happy that you went!

5. Mini-Challenges

Long-term challenges can seem unreachable, so they are hard, it's easier to make mini-challenges. 30-Day challenges are just the right length to push yourself out of your comfort zone but not be miserable. My first challenge? I gave up T.V during the week for a month! Cheers to me!

6. No-No Drawers

If you have kids, it's difficult not having some sweets and junk food in the house. The best way to keep you from getting caught with your hand in the cookie jar is to give them a designated spot that is not out in the open. Perhaps their own cabinet (not in the normal pantry) or their own drawer. You want them someplace that if you go to grab something, you're not forced to see them. Remember, out of sight, out of mind.

THE BIG PICTURE

Setting a specific goal is an effective weight-loss strategy. However, be careful not to focus on a single milestone. If your goal is slimming down because you are going on a cruise, what happens when you return? Set permanent goals, too, such as living longer, better sex or even to feel more comfortable in your clothes.

PROGRESS NOTES

Review all of the tips and tricks in this chapter. As you read them, you may have thought, "That's a great idea!" The key is to actually do them.

- Bond with your scale and use a tape measure – keeping track is motivating and will get you back on track quickly if pounds and inches reappear.

- Food Tracking Diary, Meal Plans and a "No-No" drawer. Plan what you are going to eat, and you are less likely to eat the wrong things.

- Have a Diet BFF and Go Public. Being accountable is a great recipe for success.

- Set Action Goals and Mini-Challenges. All this talk is great, but you need to plan what you will DO and make goals that aren't too overwhelming.

- Some good motivational tools? Write an email to yourself, keep Before and After photos, and make a contract with yourself.

- Be sure to stand up for yourself, even when others complain about all the nutritious food. Your body, your life, your rules.

Sylvia Williams

CHAPTER
10

GET REWARDED
PRESCRIPTION

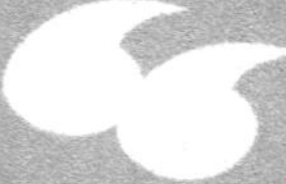

"For every disciplined effort, there is a multiple reward."

Jim Rohn

Sylvia Williams

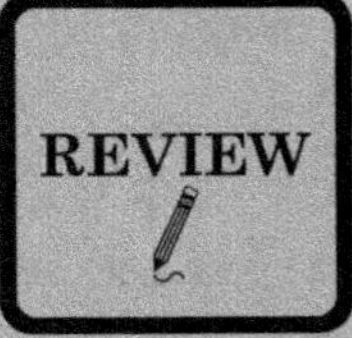

REVIEW

"I was at the end of my rope after having been a member of every, and I mean every fitness club around. Yo-yo dieting, pills and shakes, you name it, and I've done it with NO results.

I saw they were having a challenge and I thought to myself, "I can do anything for 4 weeks", and so I did.

I've already lost 40 lbs so far after deciding to stay on for the longer program! I did not expect to get what I received from Coach Syl and the program like the nutritional information, the various workouts and all of the accountability and best yet, the total support."

—Client

Do rewards help you stay focused on your weight loss journey?

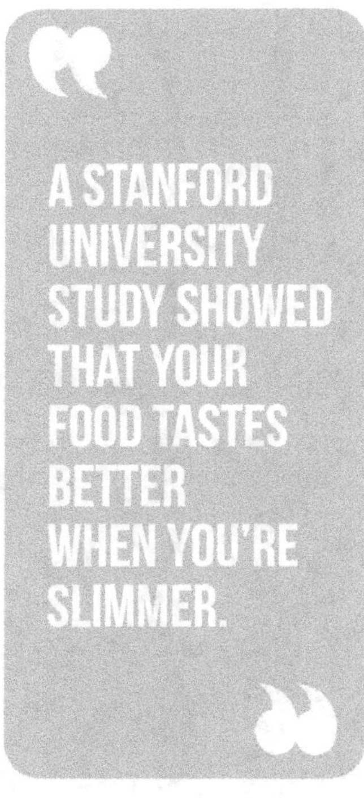

The moment I saw the ad for the Carbon 38 Sports Bra and Legging I knew I had to have them. Up to that point my "Why" had been my only driving force for reaching my goal. As explained in Chapter 1, your *Why* will evolve over time as mine had. By the time I reached my goal, I had a collection of four Why's that carried me to the finish line.

However, I discovered another powerful Prescription along the way, rewards. Rewards, like "Gold stars affixed to homework sheets, a bonus at work for a job well done, or a race medal handed to you at the finish line. It's obvious: We're hardwired to work for rewards."

I once made a public announcement to my clients in our Facebook group that I was going to reward myself with a new workout outfit once I hit my goal. As I typed the words, I could feel my knees shaking beneath the table. It was sort of a big deal. Up to that point, I was pretty casual about sharing my goals with my clients, but as I explained in the Tattle-Tale Prescription, there is power in sharing goals with clients and patients.

Without a second thought, I hit the enter button and before my eyes were the shiny 2-piece slightly risque workout gear starring back at me from my computer screen.

It didn't really help that the model in the photo didn't appear to have an ounce of fat on her body. What was I thinking? Immediately, I began to experience "Posting Regret." I expect you've heard of that. It's when you post something on social media, and then you regret it!

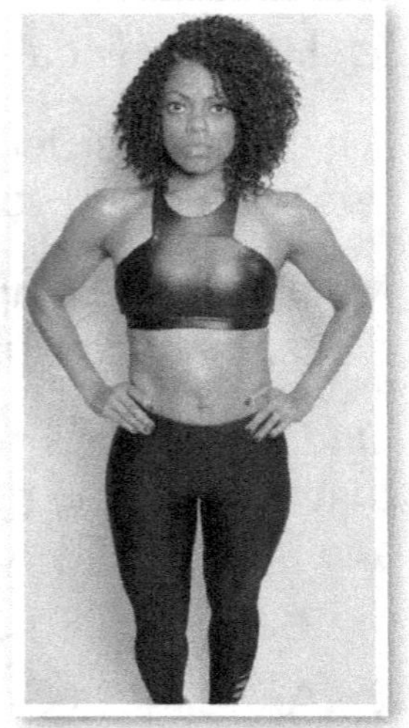

Sure, I could have deleted the post and brushed it off as a moment of temporary insanity, but there was this pinch of excitement growing in my belly. I knew that by committing to the world, well not quite the world but my small world, that I was going to pay a small fortune for this two-piece suit that would hold my feet to the fire and I was going to either fold or forge forward.

As you can see in the photo, I forged ahead, and boy did it feel good!

A Stanford University study showed that your food tastes better when you're slimmer. Sex gets better, too, report researchers at Duke University Medical Center. They found that a 10 percent loss of body weight caused increased sexual satisfaction. Also, your cognitive skills can improve, suggests a study in the Journal of *Neurology*. The point? Your body rewards you in many ways when you lose weight.

If you're on a weight loss journey, some milestone achievement rewards along the way can help keep you motivated.

Here is my prescription for cool reward suggestions for your weight loss.

Discover a fitness program worth rewarding yourself for.

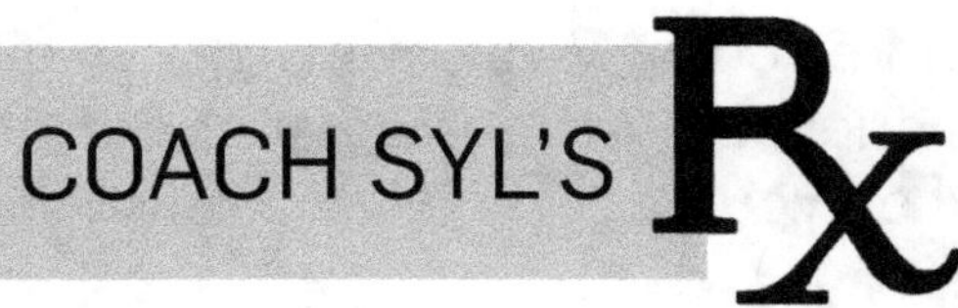

COACH SYL'S R**x**

1. Healthy Meal Service

A healthy meal delivery service can help you out for a week or two when your work schedule gets uber-busy.

Meal delivery competition is heating up with meals and ingredients that show up on your doorstep.

One service has added a new twist. They customize meals that contain the right amount of calories, carbs, healthy fats and protein for your body.

2. A Wellness Getaway

As a grand finale reward treat yourself to a vacation. Select one that is centered on health and wellness. A 2015 study from Cornell University found that experiences bring you greater, longer-lasting happiness than material things.

Book a vacation that includes activities like hiking, cycling, and other fun adventures that you might have shied away from when you were overweight.

I planned a vacation to Costa Rica for my husbands birthday, but it quickly turned into my weight loss journey completion reward. Oops ;)

3. Workout Clothes

It's a struggle to buy and wear clothes while you're losing weight. It's not realistic to fork out a hundred bucks for a new pair of designer jeans each time you drop a size. Workout clothes, on the other hand, don't need to be form-fitting and high-quality yoga pants while you're shedding pounds. Plus, being comfortable and looking good are two terrific incentives to keep going.

4. A High-speed Blender

Blenders and food processors keep getting better. Treat yourself to a Ninja blender/food processing system. It chops, grinds, purees, liquifies and makes snow cones and smoothies faster than you can say, "Yum-Yum."

5. Kitchen Scale

You'll be surprised how much bigger your eyes are than your stomach, especially when it comes to food portions. A kitchen scale helps you accurately weigh your food, so you don't consume an 8-ounce sweet potato that your eyes thought was just four ounces.

This was a great prize for our Little Black Dress Challenge winners.

6. A Bike

Remember the thrill of getting a new bike when you were a kid? Give yourself a road bike as a weight loss reward, and use it to lose even more weight!

7. Cooking Classes

When you're losing weight, it's easy to get into a chicken breast rut. Plus, how many ways can you dress up a salad? Cooking classes are a super fun way to try new, marvelous, healthy meals.

8. Pedicure

Pedicures are one of the most enjoyable reward ideas for anybody whose feet have been involved in a weight loss journey. Cosmetics aside, a pedicure can moisturize your feet and help prevent them from cracking.

9. Celebration Party

Throw yourself a weight-loss milestone party, serve sparkling apple cider and healthy appetizers and invite everyone you love. A party gives you a chance to celebrate and be congratulated. Plus, you'll be a lot less likely to fall off the wagon when everyone is aware of your journey.

10. Fitness Journal

Dozens of studies show that tracking the food you eat can help you achieve your weight goals. Dieters lost twice as much weight when they used a food journal, compared to those who didn't.

11. Massage

Reward your body and mind with a relaxing massage. In addition to feeling great, massages can improve your blood flow and relieve sore muscles. Massages can also lower blood pressure, help prevent colds, and enhance skin tone.

12. Food Chopper

The next best thing to a sous chef is the 6 in 1 Wyattnot Cutter. It chops all of your vegetables in record time. I think I use mine every day. To sweeten the pot, it even comes with a personal recipe book. You can take a shortcut by going to https://goo.gl/yFNTWp to get yours.

13.   Personal Water Bottle

Using your own special water container makes chugging water throughout the day much easier. Whether you work in a hospital, clinic or travel to visit patients, this is a health saver. It helps you stay hydrated and increases your metabolic rate by an astounding 30%!

14.   Playlist or Music Subscription

Music can offset tired feelings and increase your endurance, according to research from Brunel University's School of Sport and Education. One caveat: The music has to be between 120 to 140 beats per minute to be effective.

15.   Comedy Show

LOL lowers our stress levels, improves short-term memory and delays the storage of fat. That's no joke! So, reward your-self by snapping up some comedy tickets. P.S. When you are laughing, your abs are exercised from the contraction, and expansion of your stomach muscles.

16.   Cookbook

If it has been a while since you last bought a cookbook, you are in for a treat. There are dozens of healthy-conscious cook-books on the market today. Also, there are hundreds of free step-by-step video recipes. Google, *free video recipes.*

17.   Yoga Mat

When you reach a weight loss benchmark why not reward yourself with a new yoga mat? Yoga can be a healthy way to thank your body for putting up with years of neglect.

PROGRESS NOTES

- Rewards for milestone achievements help you stay focused on your weight loss journey

- Review the reward suggestions in this chapter and pick the ones you like. You may even think of some other rewards on your own.

- Make a list of your milestone goals and decide which reward you will give yourself for each one. You determine what the rewards are, and what you have to do to earn them

- You can even post this list in a place where you will see it daily.

- Remember to use accountability too, and post to your social media about the reward you are working towards.

Sylvia Williams

It was the last week of the eighth grade and some friends, and I were sitting on the bleachers in the gym sharing thoughts about what we were going to do in high school. I remember announcing that I planned to be the Student Council President.

And true to my word I began my freshman year of high school by joining the student council as a representative. I also joined the school newspaper staff, Future Leaders of America and other clubs that I thought were prestigious and made be appear smart.

Ironically, the more I tried to develop an egghead image, the worse my grade got. I am ashamed to say that I had no interest in academics. I just wanted to become a diet and fitness coach, and I did. However, there was a big problem.

As I became successful at helping people lose weight and improve their health, I was not following my own advice. Gradually, the weight piled on and my clothes got tighter. I was embarrassed and felt so humiliated that I didn't want to walk into the gym and have my clients see me.

Then, came a wake-up call. I received an email from a client that read, "What You Eat in Private You Wear in Public." My jaw hit the floor! I thought, 'My secret was out.' That email message should have knocked me into the real world. However, there was a problem, and its name was Sylvia.

Despite that recent reality jolt, I still was not sufficiently inspired to change my ways. Sound familiar? In desperation, I turned to prayer and asked God to give me the strength to do the right thing.

Several days and hundreds of prayers later, I awoke one rainy morning with a start. "No more," I said out loud. And that was that. I promised God that I would practice what I preach. I dropped the ugly fat I had gained and became fit again. I was transformed.

People often ask me what inspired my transformation. I tell them it occurred when I discovered the many reasons "why" I should be healthy.

I hope this book inspires you to BEGIN a life of integrity. Those of us that help people with their health have a responsibility to be a living billboard for those things we promote and stand for.

I love working with women like you, high achievers who make a contribution every day. It must be a special feeling for you to do your job and to know that you make a difference. A part of doing my job well is being a living inspiration for my clients. For that reason, I am humbled by your trust in me to help you on your journey to make a difference for yourself.

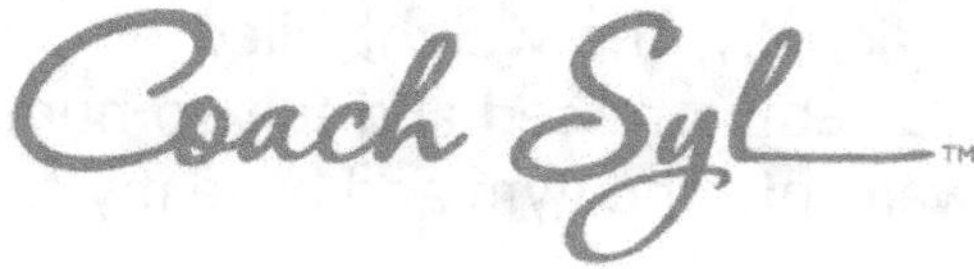

Coach Syl is a holistic nutrition coach, lifestyle entrepreneur, author, and speaker. Having achieved a successful career as a Zumba instructor, she later sought a certification as a fitness trainer in various other workout programs. After astoundingly losing nearly 50 lbs., her passion for healthy living grew and eventually introduced her to the Holistic Lifestyle, a concept that both she and her husband live by. Syl hosts the Coach Syl Show, which can be found on her Facebook page and YouTube channel. She is also a health and fitness writer with comprehensive and extensive blogs and journals followed by masses of inspired fitness advocates.

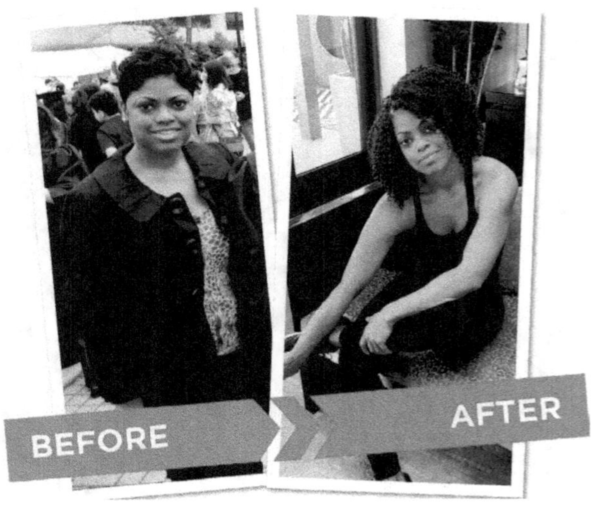

Book Coach Syl as your Keynote Speaker and You're Guaranteed to Make Your Event Highly Entertaining and Totally Unforgettable!

For nearly a decade, Syl has been encouraging and motivating people to take control of their health, bodies, and lives by changing their relationship with food.

Her origin story includes her moment of truth, and the path that led her to become the authority in helping women discover their "WHY" to transform their lives, health, relationships and of course their bodies.

After successfully building a fitness club and choosing to incorporate custom weight-loss programs over the traditional plug and play programs most gyms offer she eventually launched her online weight-loss program to have a greater reach and help transform more lives through her book, message, challenges, and online programs. Coach Syl can share relevant, actionable strategies that women can use - even if they're struggling to get started on their weight loss journey.

Her unique style inspires, empowers and entertains audiences while giving them the tools and strategies they need and want to discover their *Why*, lose the fat and gain their confidence back.

For more info, visit coachsyl.com/speaking

If you enjoyed this book or found it worthwhile, I'd be very grateful if you would post a short review on Amazon. Your support makes a difference. I read all the reviews, so I can make this book even better

Thanks again for your support!

Get in touch with me for help with any of the matters discussed in this book.

www.ingramcontent.com/pod-product-compliance
Lightning Source LLC
Chambersburg PA
CBHW051747250726
48659CB00001B/290